Lectin Free Diet

Healthy Foods from another Point of View with Recipes and Weekly Menu

Igea Bardo

Copyright © 2020 Igea Bardo

All rights reserved.

The work contained herein has been produced with the intent to provide relevant knowledge and information on the topic on the topic described in the title for entertainment purposes only. While the author has gone to every extent to furnish up to date and true information, no claims can be made as to its accuracy or validity as the author has made no claims to be an expert on this topic. Notwithstanding, the reader is asked to do their own research and consult any subject matter experts they deem necessary to ensure the quality and accuracy of the material presented herein.

This statement is legally binding as deemed by the Committee of Publishers Association and the American Bar Association for the territory of the United States. Other jurisdictions may apply their own legal statutes. Any reproduction, transmission or copying of this material contained in this work without the express written consent of the copyright holder shall be deemed as a copyright violation as per the current legislation in force on the date of publishing and subsequent time thereafter. All additional works derived from this material may be claimed by the holder of this copyright.

The data, depictions, events, descriptions and all other information forthwith are considered to be true, fair and accurate unless the work is expressly described as a work of fiction. Regardless of the nature of this work, the Publisher is exempt from any responsibility of actions taken by the reader in conjunction with this work. The Publisher acknowledges that the reader acts of their own accord and releases the author and Publisher of any responsibility for the observance of tips, advice, counsel, strategies and techniques that may be offered in this volume.

Introduction

Congratulations on purchasing *Lectin Diet: Healthy Foods from another Point of View with Recipes and Weekly Menu* by Igea Bardo, and thank you for doing so.

The following chapters will discuss the Lectin Free diet and how beneficial it will be to you. This diet will show you why you should consume foods that do not contain the compound lectin and just how good this diet will be for you. Lectin is a protein that is found in many of the foods that we consume regularly and, in plants, it is a deterrent to predators. Lectin in plants wounds or kills the insects that try to eat the plant. If it is doing that to an insect, imagine what large quantities of lectins are doing inside of your body.

The Plant Paradox diet will show you how to avoid the lectin in food and begin your journey to a life free of lectin poisoning that will lead you to a life free from gut disturbances, excess weight, skin irritations, joint pain, and other assorted inflammations.

The diet was originally developed by a cardiologist who saw daily examples of how bad diet negatively affect the human body, especially the cardiovascular system that is so important to basic life. Of all the things you might be able to live without in your life, a healthy heart is not one of them. So he developed this lectin-free diet to teach us how to rid our bodies of the toxins caused by lectins and to enable people to live longer, healthier lives.

There are many of these types of books on this subject that are available on the market today, so thanks again for choosing this one! Every effort was made to ensure it is full of as much useful information as possible, please enjoy!

Chapter 1
Lectin Free Diet: The Plant Paradox Diet

The Lectin Free is a diet plan that is gaining favor in ever-growing circles. The theory behind the Plant Paradox diet is that certain substances that are found in foods, particularly in plant-based foods, are actually poisonous to your body and will cause more harm to you than they will help you.

People who follow a plant-based diet consume only plant-based foods. They firmly believe that eating this way will allow them to lose weight and become more healthy. The Plant Paradox diet does rely on some plant-based foods, but it also eliminates many foods that carry the compounds that are harmful to your body. The Plant Paradox diet allows you to eat plenty of fresh, flavorful meals that will make you feel and look good without loading your body with those things that will add to your weight gain and inflammation.

On the Plant Paradox diet, you will eat fruits and vegetables, healthy starches, healthy fats, and good quality protein. The difference between this and other eating plans is that you will be eliminating the types of produce and starches that contain lectins. The lectins that are found in your food are bad for you for one specific reason: they are toxins. These compounds are in plants to repel animals and pests and keep them from eating the plants. When you eat these plants, you are consuming these toxins. Human beings are better able than many species to tolerate the effects of lectin, but humans eat so many foods that contain lectins that their bodies are literally loaded with this health-threatening toxin.

When you remove the plants from your diet that are full of lectins, your body will eventually cleanse itself of these toxins, and you will begin to feel better. Lectins are a highly inflammatory substance in the human body, and eliminating them will eliminate a good deal of the inflammation you are feeling. You may see weight loss immediately because tissues that are inflamed hold fluid, so reducing the inflammation will release fluid which will lead to an initial weight loss.

The lectins that are present in the food that you currently eat are blocking the receptors in your body that let your muscles burn the sugar in your blood to use for fuel. When your body is not properly using your blood glucose (sugar) for fuel, that same glucose will become stored fat in your body, beginning in the midsection. When you eliminate foods that contain lectin from your diet, these receptors will reopen, and this will allow your muscles to utilize the glucose your body makes from its food. A side benefit to this is that, when your body is properly nourished, food cravings will disappear. Your body craves food because it is missing vital nutrients, and it is prodding you to overeat so that it can search for the nutrients it needs. When you eliminate lectins and feed your body properly, food cravings will disappear. And because your body is using the blood glucose, the level of glucose in your body will automatically lessen, and your metabolism will dramatically increase. This will happen after the initial water weight loss has happened, so now you will be losing real body fat. Stabilizing your blood sugar levels and losing weight will help to lower or eliminate the risk for developing type 2 diabetes, and can help to eliminate the disease if you already have it.

Food is broken down in your digestive tract, where it becomes blood sugar to fuel your body. Your digestive system also helps to protect your body by blocking harmful substances from breaking through its walls and infecting your body. If this protective barrier is compromised in any way the walls of your intestines will loosen and allow toxins and bacteria to pass from your intestines into your bloodstream. This is known as leaky gut syndrome. When your intestines are working correctly, and the walls are strong, they will prevent toxins from passing through to the bloodstream, and the toxins and bacteria will be eliminated through waste. When leaky gut happens, those toxins and bacteria are allowed to leak out, and lectins are one of those toxins that are allowed to leak into your blood. Allowing these bacteria and viruses into your body will seriously compromise your immune system and cause more inflammation. When you eliminate the lectins from your diet, you will eliminate a major cause of leaky gut syndrome, which will then eliminate a major cause of a weakened immune system. Improving the health of your immune system will help to improve or cure certain autoimmune diseases such as thyroid disease and rheumatoid arthritis. Your belly fat, chronic fatigue, and body aches and pains will eventually disappear.

Lectins are a type of protein that is found in many of the foods that people eat on a daily basis. They are prominent especially in legumes and grains. In the human body, lectins bind themselves to the carbohydrates (carbs) in your body, especially to the sugars. As they travel through your body, they cause inflammatory or toxic reactions, and they can even interrupt the messages that must travel from one cell to another so that your body will function properly. Lectins also resist the process of digestion, and they may be responsible for interfering with your body's proper absorption of important proteins, minerals, and vitamins. When you consume those foods that are higher in lectin, then your body might not be getting the benefit of the nutrients from the other food that you eat. The top nutrients that lectin can prevent your body from absorbing are zinc, phosphorus, iron, and calcium.

Because the human body does not digest lectins, it can develop antibodies that will work to resist the lectins, treating them as foreign objects, much like a bacteria or a virus. When this happens, your responses to the foods will change. When your gut or your immune system becomes injured by the foods you eat, and your body develops antibodies against these foods, then these foods can cause an allergic-like reaction when you eat them. Allergic responses to food range from stomach aches to joint pain and stiffness to skin rashes. So when your body reacts to certain foods unfavorably, then your body will become more compromised every time you eat those foods. It would make sense that the recognized top eight allergens – fish, shellfish, soy, wheat, tree nuts, peanuts, egg, and dairy – contain some of the highest levels of lectin out of all the foods that are available to us.

Any new change in your dietary habits will be an adjustment. But opting to use the Plant Paradox diet will be the best choice you have ever made when it comes to your health and wellbeing. When you have cleared your body of the harmful substance lectin, when you have removed the toxins and inflammatories from your body, you will begin to realize how good the food that you eat can make you feel. And that is the primary goal of the Plant Paradox diet.

Chapter 2
Plant Friends And Plant Enemies

Lectin is a protein in your food that will cause many adverse effects on your body.

But there is another protein that you should also steer clear of, and that is the A1 Protein.

Milk is full of proteins, and the largest group of milk proteins is the group known as casein. This protein is a dairy protein that is slow to digest in the human body. The two major forms of casein in dairy milk are the A1 beta-casein and the A2 beta-casein. Evidence has begun to point out that the A1 protein is more of a harmful protein and should not be ingested by anyone with lactose intolerance. The A1 protein is actually a mutation of the A2 protein and is thought to be linked to many chronic health problems in humans, such as digestive issues, heart disease, and diabetes. A1 is one of the lectin compounds that you need to avoid.

Lectins are considered to be antinutrients, because they work against the nutrients that your body needs to absorb and prevents you from absorbing them. One of the worst lectins that you can consume is the wheat germ, which is found in the seeds of the wheat family and in wheat itself. Gluten is a part of the wheat germ, and while the negative effects from gluten are not considered to be as bad as those from wheat germ, gluten is still a lectin that you need to avoid for optimum health.

One major way that lectins will harm your body is through a process called molecular mimicry. The lectins will mimic, or pretend to be, the same as the proteins in your joints or in your thyroid gland, which then causes your body to attack itself, trying to rid itself of inflammation.

You will want to avoid all foods that contain lectin if you want to enjoy a life free from pain, inflammation, and chronic disease. There are many foods that you will want to avoid, but most of them fall into three main categories that are legumes, nightshade vegetables, and grains. Here are the foods that you will want to avoid when you are on the lectin-free diet as they are among the highest for levels of lectins.

SQUASHES. The squash family is native to America. This includes all fruit that has a peel and grows on a vine, which is the butternut squash, zucchini, acorn squash, and pumpkins. Cucumbers are also part of this family, but they originated in Asia. Besides being full of lectins, the squash family of foods also contains various sugars that will send messages to your body, telling it to store fat for future needs.

DAIRY. Any dairy product that comes from cows in North America will have the A1 protein, which must be avoided. This is true even for milk that comes from cows that are organically raised and fed with grass instead of feed. You may drink cow's milk that comes from cows in Southern Europe as well as water buffalo milk, sheep's milk, and goat's milk. You can use coconut milk, both canned and the kind that comes in cartons in the refrigerated section, to replace milk in any recipe.

BEANS AND LEGUMES -- Legumes, also known as pulses, are the foods such as lentils, soybeans, peas, and beans. This group has the highest content of lectins out of any food group. There is no secret why beans are known for causing indigestion, bloating, and gas.

VEGETABLE OILS -- Vegetable oils are made from the same foods that are high in lectins, like sunflowers, soybeans, and corn. And most of these oils are made from plants that have been modified genetically, which means that they are specially bred to contain more lectins to repel more insects. And the fats that are found in these oils are the inflammation-producing omega-6 fatty acid variety and not the healthy omega-3 kind.

MEAT THAT IS RAISED BY CONVENTIONAL METHODS -- Corn is full of lectin. Corn is used to feed cows. The by-products of the corn that the cows eat end up in your body as lectins. And corn will cause fat deposits to collect in your muscles.

THE NIGHTSHADES -- While many different theories abound as to why the nightshades are called nightshades, the thing that you need to remember is that the nightshades are full of lectin. This includes tomatoes, goji berries, eggplants, hot peppers, bell peppers, and potatoes.

QUINOA -- This grain-like substance is lauded as a gluten-free substitution for grains that contain gluten, the fact that it is so full of lectins means that it will not be helpful for your waistline, immune system, or your digestive tract.

CORN -- This is considered to be a vegetable, but it is really a grain. It is full of lectin. And because corn is one of the largest crops that is grown and since corn is found in so many other products as a food additive – think of corn chips, corn-based breakfast cereals like cornflakes, cornstarch, corn syrup – the average American diet is loaded with corn.

CASHEWS AND PEANUTS -- These two popular foods are not nuts but rather legumes and they are full of lectins. The shell that covers the cashew is so toxic to humans that people must wear gloves when they harvest and process cashews. Peanuts are also full of lectin.

The idea behind the Plant Paradox diet program is to remove the lectins from your diet that is causing the inflammation in your body. This will allow your body to get nutrients from good, lectin-free foods and begin to heal itself. So the general list of foods that you will want to avoid when you are on the Plant Paradox diet is as follows:

- Cow's milk and cow's milk products which includes cheese, cottage cheese, yogurt, and ice cream
- Seeds and nuts like sunflower seeds, pumpkin seeds, chia seeds, cashews, and peanuts
- Vegetables that have beans or seeds in them like sugar snap peas and green beans
- Fruits that are usually referred to as vegetables like eggplant, melons, bell peppers, hot peppers, all squashes, tomatoes, and cucumbers
- Any food that contains soy like tofu, edamame, soy sauce, and soy milk
- Legumes, such as peas, chickpeas, lentils, soybeans, kidney beans, black beans, navy beans, and pinto beans

- Any form of grain which includes all forms of flour, refined grains, whole grains, and any form of corn, corn product, oats, and rice

When you are beginning any eating plan that is designed to improve your health and wellbeing, you will hear many different references to the words macronutrients and micronutrients. While these words may sound daunting, they really aren't. Micronutrients, or micros, are simply the antioxidants, minerals, and vitamins that you get from the food that you eat. Macronutrients, or macros, are the three large groups of food that you eat every day, your proteins, carbs, and fats. As long as you are eating a balanced diet with all three of the macros, then you will easily get all of the micros that you need.

Chapter 3
Shopping For The Plant Paradox Diet

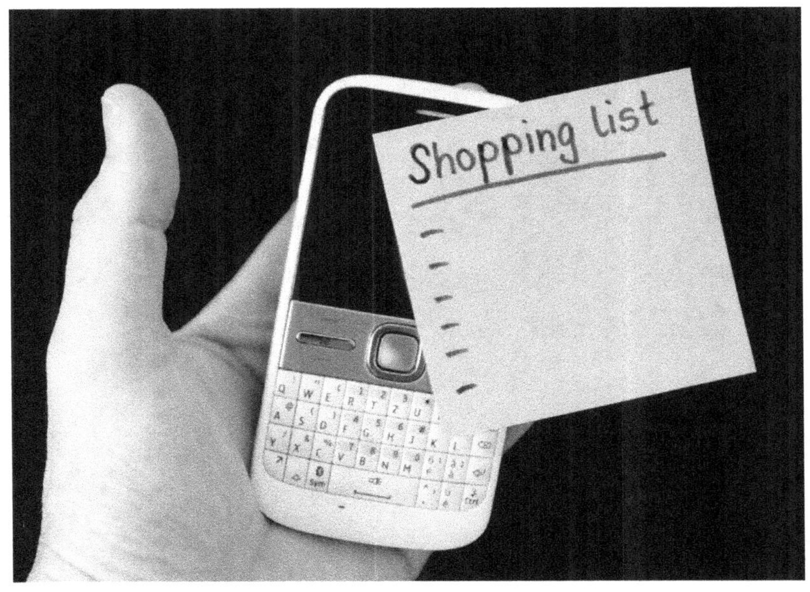

The first step in beginning to follow the Plant Paradox diet is to buy the foods that are low in lectin that will allow you to make the healthy meals that your body is craving. When you allow lectins to invade your body, they will cause more harm than good. They will give you health issues like brain fog, weight gain, leaky gut syndrome, skin rashes, and problems with inflammation. So as long as you purchase the proper, low-lectin foods to use when planning your meals, then you will be well prepared for living lectin-free and healthy. Here are the foods that you will be consuming on the Lectin Free diet.

FOODS TO EAT ON THE PLANT PARADOX DIET

VEGETABLES – Mushrooms, seaweed, algae, purslane, mint, basil, parsley, mizuna, mustard greens, escarole, butter lettuce, fennel, dandelion greens, endive, spinach, kohlrabi, red leaf lettuce, green leaf lettuce, romaine lettuce, leafy greens, asparagus, okra, hearts of palm, cilantro, artichokes, radishes, beets, carrots, carrot greens, chicory, scallions, chives, leeks, onions, celery, green cabbage, red cabbage, kale, collards, watercress, arugula, Swiss chard, Chinese cabbage, bok choy, cauliflower, and Brussels sprouts.

FRUITS – Avocado, raspberries, mulberries, blueberries, blackberries, strawberries.

FISH – Anchovies, sardines, mussels, oysters, calamari, squid, scallops, lobster, crab, shrimp, halibut, tuna in cans, tuna fillets, salmon, freshwater bass, white fish.

DIARY PRODUCTS – Organic cream cheese, organic sour cream, organic heavy cream, coconut yogurt, plain sheep cheese, goat kefir, sheep kefir, goat cheese, goat butter, A2 milk, and butter made from the milk of grass-fed cows, French or Italian cheeses, organic cream cheese, any cheese from Switzerland, buffalo butter, ghee, organic heavy cream, organic sour cream.

SEEDS AND NUTS –Brazil nuts, pine nuts, psyllium, hemp protein powder, sesame seeds, hemp seeds, flaxseeds, chestnuts, hazelnuts, coconut, pecans, pistachios, walnuts, and macadamia nuts

OILS – Cod liver oil, sesame oil, rice bran oil, red palm oil, walnut oil, perilla oil, avocado oil, MCT oil, macadamia oil, coconut oil, olive oil, and algae oil

SWEETENERS – Xylitol, Erythritol, monk fruit, yacon, inulin, and stevia

FLOURS – Arrowroot, grape seed, tiger nut, sweet potato, green banana, cassava, chestnut, sesame, hazelnut, almond, and coconut

SEASONINGS AND HERBS – All are allowed except for flaked chili peppers; miso is also allowed

RESISTANT STARCHES – In moderation -- Rutabaga, sweet potato, yam, cassava, baobab fruit, green bananas, green plantains, and coconut flakes cereal, bagels and bread made with coconut flour

PLANT-BASED MEATS – Tempeh, veggie burger, Hilary root, hemp tofu, Quorn

PASTURED-RAISED POULTRY – NOT farm-raised -- Grouse, dove, quail, duck, pasteurized eggs, ostrich, turkey, chicken

MEAT – Grass-fed – Elk, venison, wild game, bison, beef, lamb, pork

MISCELLANEOUS – Shirataki noodles, champagne (one six-ounce glass per day), red wine (one six-ounce glass per day), aged spirits (one ounce per day), dark chocolate (seventy-two percent or higher), all types of olives, keto fat bombs, coconut ice cream, dairy and sugar-free frozen desserts

Most of these foods can be found in your local grocery store, big-box retailer, or specialty foods store, wherever you shop regularly. You can also find some of these foods online if you want to buy them in bulk quantities, things like your seasonings, flours, and nuts and seeds. Look at a butcher shop or seafood shop for allowable meat and fish because often these stores are not much more expensive than a regular grocery store. You will want to source your fruits from local sources like smaller grocery stores, roadside stands, and farmer's markets, because most fruit is off-limits unless it is in season when the levels of lectins in the fruit are lower. Here is a list of fruits and the season in which they are considered to be 'in season' so that you will be able to enjoy them occasionally:

SPRING FRUITS – Artichoke, strawberries, rhubarb, pineapple, mango, avocado, and apricots

SUMMER – Watermelon, raspberries, plums, peaches, nectarines, blueberries, blackberries

AUTUMN – Pomegranate, pears, grapes, figs, cranberries, apples

WINTER – Tangerines, oranges, lemons, grapefruit, chestnuts

If the fruit is not on the list and not in season, then you must avoid eating it because it will be full of lectins. As you can see, many of your meals will be based around vegetables, with other items added in or used as sides. It is important to eat only these foods that are low in lectins or have no lectins at all. Equally important is the list of foods that you will not eat, the foods you will need to avoid.

FOODS TO AVOID ON THE PLANT PARADOX DIET

VEGETABLES AND FRUITS – Goji berries, eggplant, melons, squashes, pumpkin, zucchini, ripe bananas, all fruits except for the ones that are in season.

You may not eat chili peppers, bell peppers, or tomatoes unless they are peeled and deseeded.

COW'S MILK PRODUCTS – those made from cows not from Southern Europe – Casein protein powders, kefir, cottage cheese, ricotta, American cheese, frozen yogurt, Greek yogurt, any dairy product that contain A1 protein.

OILS – Partially hydrogenated canola or vegetable oil, sunflower oil, safflower oil, cottonseed oil, peanut oil, corn oil, grapeseed oil, and soy oil.

GRASSES, SPROUTED GRAINS, PSEUDO GRAINS – Barley grass, wheatgrass, popcorn, corn syrup, cornstarch, corn products, corn, spelt, buckwheat, kasha, barley, white rice, brown rice, bulgur, rye, quinoa, oats, wheat Kamut, wheat einkorn, and whole grains.

SEEDS AND NUTS – Cashews, peanuts, chia seeds, sunflower seeds, pumpkin seeds

REFINED STARCHY FOODS – Maltodextrin, diet drinks, sugar substitutes, agave, sugar, cereal, crackers, cookies, flours made from grains ad pseudo-grains, pastry, tortillas, bread, milk, potato chips, potatoes, rice, and pasta.

ANY FORM OF soybean fed or grain-fed pork, lamb, beef, poultry, shellfish, or fish

So when you make your shopping list and begin to buy your foods to make your lectin-free meals, just take this list with you and only buy the foods that are listed as safe to eat. After a few weeks on the Plant Paradox diet, you will wonder why those high-lectin foods ever appealed to you. You will feel so much better when you eliminate the lectins and their toxins from your daily diet that you will wonder why you have not been living this way all along.

Chapter 4
How The Plant Paradox Diet Works

Since you have decided to make the change to healthier living by beginning the Plant Paradox diet, the time to begin is now. You will not begin to enjoy a healthier life until you start so don't put it off any longer. It is time to eliminate from your life the lectins that cause damage to your gut, interrupt your normal digestive processes, and cause deficiencies in the nutrients your body needs so desperately. There are several stages to the Plant Paradox diet and you will want to follow all of the stages in order so that you will have the best foundation for cleansing your body and eliminating lectins from your diet.

PREPARE YOUR BODY FOR HEALTHY EATING – PHASE ONE

The very first thing that you will need to do when you begin the Plant Paradox diet is to prepare your body for healthy eating. You have probably been living on a diet of lectins and processed foods and sugars for years, and the unhealthy bacteria that normally live in small amounts in your gut have taken over and made you feel fat, bloated, and irregular. These bad bacteria will also cause you to feel cravings for more bad foods and give you a non-stop appetite. If you have ever eaten something and then eaten something else and something else because what you are eating truly is not satisfying your appetite, then you are probably feeling the effects of toxins that come from lectins.

When you change your diet the will heal your gut and the bad bacteria will eventually subside back to the levels they are supposed to be as the good bacteria are revived and once again restore the health of your gut. Then you will begin to lose weight and the levels of inflammation in your body will decrease. To prepare your body for the benefits of the Plant Paradox diet the first thing you will need to do is to cleanse your body, and you will do that by using a detoxifying three-day cleanse to restore health to your gut.

The three-day cleanse is designed to kick start your lectin-free lifestyle. This cleanse will work to change the types of bacteria that are currently living in your gut and causing you harm. Once you do this cleanse then it will be imperative that you begin on the Plant Paradox diet immediately so that you do not lose any of the progress you have made.

To begin the three-day cleanse you will completely eliminate from your diet the following foods:

Dairy	Grains	Pseudo-grains
Fruit	Sugar	Seeds
Eggs	Soy	Nightshade plants
Roots	Tubers	Corn
Inflammatory oils	Farm animal proteins	

You may be wondering what you will be eating. The first three days will be filled with good, healthy foods that will cleanse your body and jump start your weight loss.

You will mostly be eating healthy vegetables from this list:

Broccoli	Brussels sprouts	Cauliflower
Bok choy	Napa cabbage	Chinese cabbage
Swiss chard	Arugula	Watercress
Collards	Kale	Cabbage
Radicchio	Raw sauerkraut	Kimchi
Celery	Onions	Leeks
Chives	Scallions	Chicory
Carrots	Carrot greens	Artichokes
Beets	Radishes	Artichokes
Hearts of palm	Cilantro	Okra
Asparagus	Garlic	Leafy greens
Romaine	Kohlrabi	Spinach
Endive	Dandelion greens	Butter lettuce
Fennel	Escarole	Mustard greens
Parsley	Basil	Mint
Purslane	Perilla	Algae
Seaweed	Mushrooms	Sea vegetables*

*Sea vegetables include alaria, bladderwrack, ogonori, sea lettuce, luminaria japonica, kelp, agar, dulse, hijiki, wakame, Kombu, arame.

The list of vegetables are the ones that you are allowed to eat in any quantity and either raw or cooked. These can be purchased either fresh or frozen, but make sure that you purchase them as organic.

PROTEIN – On the three-day starter cleanse you will only eat small amounts of chicken that was raised in a pasture and not grain fed, or healthy fish. But do not consume more than two four-ounce portions each day. It is best to measure your portions, but if you want a visual reference a four ounce portion of meat or fish is about the size of a deck of cards.

GOOD FATS AND OILS

Your body will get most of the good fats that it needs if you will just eat one whole avocado every day. When you are looking for healthy oils for your three-day cleanse the following are all allowed:

Flaxseed oil	Hemp seed oil	Extra virgin olive oil
Walnut oil	Sesame seed oil	Macadamia nut oil
Coconut oil	Avocado oil	

Nuts on the yes list are also allowed, but no more than one-half cup per day.

SEASONINGS, SAUCES, AND DRESSINGS

You need to avoid any sauce or dressing that is processed. You can use olive oil and fresh lemon to flavor most of the foods that you will be eating. You will also be allowed to use the following:

Fresh spices	Fresh herbs	Sea salt
Mustard	Vinegar	Fresh crack black pepper

To quench your thirst during this time you will want to rely on decaffeinated coffee, unsweetened tea, tap water, or sparkling water. You should make a goal to drink at least eight cups of these fluids every day, in addition to the fluids that you get from your foods. The cleanse might feel restrictive but it only lasts for three days and it is the jump start that your body needs in order to regain the healthy balances you have been lacking. Keep in mind that you can eat as many of the listed veggies as you need to in order to keep yourself full and satisfied. So after you finish the three-day cleanse you will be ready to begin Phase Two of the Plant Paradox program.

REPAIR AND RESTORE YOUR BODY – PHASE TWO

During Phase Two you are starting with a cleansed body and you need to make every effort to treat it right during the next six weeks. You will now be restructuring your basic eating habits so that you can retrain your body for healthy living. This will keep the healthy bacteria in your gut thriving and keep the unhealthy bacteria restrained. In Phase Two, which will last for the next six weeks, you can eat anything that you were allowed to eat in Phase One, and you can add in the following foods

In-season fruits, limited	Figs	Dates
Pastured eggs	Plantains	Shirataki noodles
Parsnips	Turnips	Jicama
Celery root	Sunchokes	Yams
Sweet potatoes	Almond flour	Cassava flour
Coconut flour	Sorghum	Millet
Inulin	Yacon syrup	Goat milk yogurt
Olives	Sheep milk yogurt	Coconut yogurt

You may also add back in casein in limited amounts, but only those products that contain the A2 protein and never the A1 protein.

REAP THE REWARDS IN PHASE THREE

This is the last phase of working the actual program before you incorporate this diet into your daily lifestyle. Keep your consumption of fruit to very low levels and only eat those fruits that are in season. Always remove the peels and seeds from the fruits that you do eat and only consume the pulp of the fruit. This is the phase where you will begin to enjoy the benefits of your hard work over the last seven weeks in the form of better looking skin and hair, clearer thinking, lessened or eliminated joint pains, weight loss, better sleep, and improved energy.

During Phase Three you will continue to eat all of the foods that you have been eating, and you will add in the following foods:

- Eggplant, zucchini, and baby cucumbers that have been peeled and the seeds removed
- White Indian basmati rice that has been cooked in a pressure cooker or an air fryer
- Organic lentils and beans that have been cooked in a pressure cooker or an air fryer
- Bell peppers and tomatoes that have been peeled and had the seeds removed
- You may add in minimal amounts of artisan white sourdough bread if you truly miss eating bread, but only one slice per day, and don't eat it if you suffer from memory loss, prediabetes, diabetes, gluten sensitivity, celiac disease, or if you have an autoimmune disorder.

These foods will need to be added back into your diet in small amounts and only add in one to test for a week, to see how they affect your body. If you do not like the way they make you feel then do not eat them.

KEEPING THE PLANT PARADOX PROGRAM FOR LIFE USING A NEW AND IMPROVED FOOD PYRAMID

Now for the remainder of your life you will be eating a healthy diet with minimal or no amounts of harmful lectins.

The bulk of your diet will still be vegetables from the approved list, especially green leafy vegetables, and healthy fats in the form of avocados and healthy oils. You can now add in intermittent fasting, which is part of the Plant Paradox diet pyramid, to accelerate your weight loss. This new pyramid that you will be using is the ultimate guide to a blueprint for healthy living.

Adding in intermittent fasting is not required but it is recommended to keep your weight loss on track and to keep your body functioning properly. Humans have been fasting for various reasons for centuries, and while going without food may seem like a big deal it really isn't. Intermittent fasting means that certain hours of the day you will eat and certain hours of the day you will not eat. The most popular of the various methods of fasting is the 16:8 rule of fasting. On this method you will consume all of the food that you eat during one eight-hour period of the day and you will not eat for the other sixteen hours of the day. What works best for most people is to schedule those eight hours of eating from eleven in the morning to seven at night, or from noon to eight in the evening. This will give you eight hours to consume food while you are going about your daily activities. The sixteen hours that you are fasting would then run from seven or eight in the evening to eleven in the morning or noon of the next day. Part of these hours you will be asleep. When you wake you are free to drink all of the decaffeinated coffee and teas that you want, along with plain water or sparkling water. Liquids do not count as breaking your fast. The hours that you are awake and not eating are really not so many that you will be bothered by them, and foregoing the consumption of food is a great way to keep your body relying on burning excess fat so you will continue to lose weight.

When you embark on the Plant Paradox diet you will probably want to add a few new small appliances to your kitchen if you do not already own them. You will want a blender and/or a food processor, a pressure cooker or an instant pot, peelers for the vegetables, and a spiralizer. You will use the spiralizer to make spiral shaped noodles out of any firm vegetable like a zucchini or a sweet potato. A microwave is also nice to have, as is an assortment of skillets and pots to cook in and mixing bowls of different sizes. A salad spinner is nice to have, so that you can rinse and dry your leafy greens and other salad ingredients, but a colander and paper towels will work just as well for this.

And you are now armed with all of the information that you need in order to begin the Plant Paradox diet.

Chapter 5
Three-Day Detox Recipes

You might be looking at the list of allowed foods on the three-day detox phase and wondering what you can do with them. Here are some recipes using the foods that are allowed to help you get started.

Certain food items like coconut milk, lemon juice, avocado oil, coconut oil, olive oil, and seasonings should be staple items in your kitchen. There will also be a notation of ingredients needed, a type of 'shopping list' for every recipe.

Green Ginger Smoothie

You can prep these in advance because this recipe makes four packets. The extras can be stored in the freezer for later use for a quick breakfast or a between-meal snack (yes, light snacking is allowed!).

<u>Shopping list</u>

Romaine or spinach, avocados, mint leaves

<u>Ingredients</u>

Romaine lettuce or spinach, chopped, four cups*

Mint leaves, one cup

Avocadoes, two

Ginger, freshly minced, two tablespoons

<u>**When you want to enjoy the smoothie add in these**</u>

<u>**ingredients**</u>

Liquid stevia, vanilla flavor, five or six drops

Lemon juice, three tablespoons

Coconut milk, unsweetened, one cup

<u>**Instructions**</u>

Mix each of four smoothie packs by placing in a freezer-safe bag one cup of the chopped spinach or romaine, one-fourth cup of the mint leaves, one half of an avocado, and one half of a tablespoon of the freshly minced ginger. These will be safe in your freezer for three months.

When you want to make a smoothie, just put one pack of ingredients into the blender along with the finishing ingredients and blend all of the ingredients together until the smoothie is creamy and smooth, then drink it immediately.

If you use the romaine lettuce, your smoothie will have a slightly more delicate taste to it than if you use the spinach, which will give the smoothie a greener, slightly bitter flavor.

Green Veggie Hash

This recipe makes a wonderful mix of onions and green veggies and is seasoned with spices before being roasted to set all of the flavors in. You can eat this by itself or with many other recipes. In Phase Two or Three, you can enjoy this recipe with an egg on top or on the side. You can make this in a large batch and store it in your refrigerator for up to four days.

This recipe will also give you a reason to use all of the stems that you have been chopping off of your leafy greens, because they are full of nutrients and should not be wasted.

This recipe will make six servings.

Shopping list

onion, asparagus, Brussels sprouts, broccoli

Ingredients

Stems from your greens, one cup diced finely

Onion, one large white, diced finely

Asparagus, two cups, trimmed, chopped into bite-size pieces

Brussels sprouts, quartered, three cups

Broccoli, diced, four cups

Paprika, one half teaspoon

Black pepper, one half teaspoon

Onion powder, one half teaspoon

Garlic powder, one teaspoon

Cumin, one teaspoon

Sea salt, one teaspoon

Rosemary, dried, two tablespoons

Avocado oil, one fourth cup

<u>**Instructions**</u>

Heat the oven to 400. Mix together in a large bowl the paprika, black pepper, onion powder, garlic powder, cumin, sea salt, rosemary, and the avocado oil until these are all blended well. Stir in the onion, stems, asparagus, Brussels sprouts, and broccoli and toss all of these ingredients gently but thoroughly until all of the veggies are well coated. Spread this mixture out on a large baking sheet, or bake it in two batches if necessary, for twenty to twenty-five minutes, until the veggies are tender and the edges have just begun to brown. You can eat this immediately or let it cool to room temperature and store it in the refrigerator for future use.

If you are in Phase Two or Three, you can serve this warm with a couple of eggs that are cooked the way you like them. If you are eating vegan, then add in a half cup of walnuts or avocado to make this dish a bit heartier.

Breakfast Salad Dressing

This dressing has a zesty citrus flavor.

<u>**Shopping list**</u>

walnut oil

<u>**Ingredients**</u>

Cumin, one fourth teaspoon

Sea salt, one teaspoon

Dijon mustard, one teaspoon

Lemon zest, one tablespoon

Lemon juice, one tablespoon

Red wine vinegar, one fourth cup

Walnut oil, one half cup

<u>**Instructions**</u>

In a large glass jar with a secure lid, put all of the ingredients and shake them together well.

Keep this dressing in your refrigerator, where it will remain fresh for up to two weeks. Shake

it well every time before you want to use it.

Breakfast Salad

Salad is great for any meal of the day, and it is so portable that you can make it in advance and take it with you to work or school. This salad isn't just a bowl of leafy greens either! This recipe makes one salad

Shopping list

mixed greens, mint leaves, avocado, broccoli

Ingredients

Mixed greens, two cups*

Mint leaves, chopped roughly, one fourth cup

Avocado, one half diced

Broccoli, chopped finely, one half cup

Green Veggie Hash, one-half cup either chilled or at room temperature

Breakfast Salad dressing, two tablespoons

Instructions

Use a large bowl to toss together the avocado, shredded broccoli, veggie hash, and the dressing until all of the ingredients of the salad are well coated with the dressing.

Mix together the salad greens with the chopped mint. Pour the hash mixture on top of the greens and enjoy.

*You can buy power mix or spring mix from the grocery store or you can make your own salad mix by combining one part kale, one part arugula, one part chopped lettuce, and one part spinach.

Nutty Green Salad

This is great for taking to work or school because you can make this salad ahead of time by coating the avocado slices with a little lemon juice to keep them from turning brown. This recipe makes one salad.

<u>Shopping list</u>

mixed greens, fresh herbs, avocado, broccoli

<u>Ingredients</u>

Mixed greens, two cups

Nutty Green Salad Dressing, two to three tablespoons

Fresh herbs, minced, one-fourth cup, use parsley, dill, tarragon, rosemary,   thyme, basil, or mint in any combination to make one fourth cup

Avocado, one half diced

Broccoli, finely shredded, one half cup

Nut mix, one fourth cup

<u>Instructions</u>

Toss together the salad dressing, nut mix, herbs, avocado, and the shredded broccoli in a large mixing bowl. Arrange your mixed greens in a bowl or a container for carrying and then arrange the slaw mix on top.

If you want to make this recipe and take it with you, it might be better to mix it in a large jar by layering the ingredients. Put the dressing on the bottom of the jar, then add in the nut mix, avocado tossed with lemon juice, shredded broccoli, herbs, and lastly the salad greens. When lunchtime arrives, just remove the lid from the jar, lay a plate over the jar, and turn the plate and the jar over to dup the salad out onto the plate. If you are in Phase Two or Three,

you can enjoy this salad with a bit of prosciutto or a salmon fillet.

Nutty Green Salad Dressing

This dressing is a bit sweet, spicy, smooth, and warm all at the same time.

Shopping list

tahini

Ingredients

Paprika, one fourth teaspoon

Sea salt, one teaspoon

Dijon mustard, one teaspoon

Tahini, one tablespoon

Balsamic vinegar, one fourth cup

Red wine vinegar, one fourth cup

Olive oil, one half cup

Instructions

Blend all of the ingredients in a glass jar and shake it well to mix all of the flavors. This will remain fresh in your refrigerator for up to two weeks, and shake it well again every time that you want to use it.

If you are following a keto meal plan, then cut the vinegars in half and doubles the olive oil.

Nut Mix

This recipe makes twelve to fifteen servings and is great eaten by itself or added to any salad recipe. It might taste like junk food, but it is very healthy and satisfying.

Shopping list

walnut oil, raw pine nuts, raw macadamia nuts, raw pecans, raw walnuts

Ingredients

Sea salt, one teaspoon

Thyme, dried, one teaspoon

Sage, dried, one tablespoon

Rosemary, dried, two tablespoons

Garlic, minced, four tablespoons

Walnut oil, two tablespoons

Pine nuts, raw, one half cup

Macadamia nuts, raw, one half cup

Pecans, raw, one cup

Walnuts, raw, two cups

Instructions

Mix the nuts together in a large size heatproof bowl and set this off to the side. Heat the walnut oil in a small skillet and place the thyme, sage, rosemary, and garlic and cook the seasonings for four or five minutes until they are well mixed and very fragrant. Stir in the sea sat and then immediately pour this over the mixed nuts in the large bowl. Toss the ingredients together well and then let it cool down to room temperature before you serve it.

This mixture will remain fresh in your refrigerator for as long as two weeks, or you can prepare it and freeze it for as long as six weeks.

Mushroom and Sage Soup

This soup is so rich and thick it will make you feel as though you are enjoying a holiday meal any time of year. If you would like the soup to be a bit lighter, then leave out the coconut milk and use water in its place or double the amount of broth.

Shopping list

vegetable broth, celery, onion, mushrooms, cauliflower

<u>Ingredients</u>

Broth, vegetable or chicken, preferably homemade

Coconut milk, unsweetened, three cups

Mustard powder, dried, one half teaspoon

Onion powder, one half teaspoon

Black pepper, one half teaspoon

Sea salt, one teaspoon

Lemon juice, one tablespoon

Thyme, dried, one teaspoon

Sage, dried, one tablespoon

Garlic, minced, two tablespoons

Celery, two ribs diced

Onion, one medium size diced

Mushrooms, two pounds, washed and dried, trimmed and diced

Cauliflower, florets, four cups

Avocado oil, three tablespoons divided

<u>Instructions</u>

Set a large pot on a medium-high heat and heat the avocado oil until it shimmers.

Pour in the celery, onion, mushrooms, and cauliflower florets and let them cook for five minutes while you stir often. Mix in the lemon juice, thyme, sage, and garlic and cook for three minutes more while you stir this constantly. Then blend in the mustard powder, onion powder, pepper, and salt and mix well for two minutes. Blend in the coconut milk and the broth and then turn the heat to simmer for thirty minutes. Carefully puree the cooked soup. Serve it immediately or allow it to come to room temperature to store.

This will remain fresh in your refrigerator for up to one week or in your freezer for three months.

Avocado and Salmon Bowl

This makes one bowl.

Shopping list

avocado, riced cauliflower, salmon

Ingredients

Nutty Green Salad Dressing, two tablespoons

Lime juice, one tablespoon

Cilantro, minced, one tablespoon

Avocado, one quarter sliced thin

Green Veggie Hash, one cup

Cauliflower Rice, one cup

Seafood Spice Rub, one teaspoon

Salmon, wild-caught, one three-ounce fillet

Avocado oil, one teaspoon

Instructions

Heat the broiler to high. Use a brush to brush some of the oil onto the bottom of a small baking dish. Use the rest of the oil to coat the salmon fillet and then sprinkle the Seafood Spice Rub on it. Lay the salmon in the baking dish with the skin side down and broil it for eight minutes. While it is broiling then heat up the Green Veggie Hash and the Cauliflower Rice, or you can leave both at room temperature. Add the Green Veggie Hash on top of the Cauliflower Rice in a serving bowl. Put the salmon fillet on top of the Green Veggie Hash and then garnish with the dressing, lime juice, and cilantro.

To make this recipe, vegan use jackfruit instead of salmon and only broil it for five minutes.

Cauliflower Rice

This makes two cups and will remain fresh in your refrigerator for up to five days.

Shopping list

yellow onion,

rice cauliflower

Ingredients

Sea salt, one half teaspoon

Cauliflower rice, twelve ounces, fresh riced or purchased frozen

Yellow onion, one minced

Olive oil, one fourth cup

Instructions

Fry the minced onion in the olive oil for three to four minutes until the onion is tender. Add in the salt and the cauliflower rice and cook for seven to ten minutes more while stirring often.

Seafood Spice Rub

This spice rub is good not only on seafood but also on pork, chicken, other fish, and even on veggies. It also works well sprinkled on eggs or stirred into soup. This is stored at room temperature and will remain fresh for up to six months.

<u>Ingredients</u>

Cloves, ground, one half teaspoon

Cinnamon, ground, one teaspoon

Curry powder, one teaspoon

Onion powder, one and one half teaspoon

Black pepper, two teaspoons

Garlic powder, one tablespoon

Cumin, one tablespoon

Paprika, ground, two tablespoons

Sea salt, two tablespoons

<u>Instructions</u>

Keep the ingredients fresh in a glass jar with a lid and shake it before each time that you use it.

Cauliflower Spinach Risotto

This is risotto made without rice that is full of color as well as flavor and is still creamy and rich. This will freeze for up to three months or remain fresh in your refrigerator for one week.

<u>Shopping list</u>

nutritional yeast, coconut cream, vegetable broth, riced cauliflower, baby spinach, shallots

<u>Ingredients</u>

Black pepper, one teaspoon

Sea salt, one teaspoon

Lemon juice, two tablespoons

Nutritional yeast, one fourth cup

Coconut cream, one thirteen to fourteen ounce can

Vegetables or chicken broth, preferably homemade, two cups

Cauliflower rice, two sixteen-ounce packages

Baby spinach, three cups packed

Garlic, minced, three tablespoons

Shallots, four minced

Avocado oil, one fourth cup

Instructions

Fry the shallots and garlic in the hot avocado oil on a medium-high heat in a large pot for making soup while you stir frequently. Drop in the spinach and cook it until it wilts. Then add in the cauliflower rice and continue frying, stirring often, until all of the liquid has disappeared. Pour in the lemon juice, nutritional yeast, coconut cream, and broth and blend them in well, letting this mixture cook until it becomes thick. Blend in the salt and pepper and serve.

Quorn Taco Salad

This spicy salad is served over lettuce instead of chips and has all of the elements of a classic taco salad. This can also be packed up to take with you.

Shopping list

nutritional yeast, mixed greens, Quorn grounds

<u>Ingredients</u>

Nutritional yeast, one fourth cup

Guacamole, one fourth cup

Taco Salad Dressing, one fourth cup

Mixed salad greens, four cups

Sea salt, one half teaspoon

Black pepper, one half teaspoon

Paprika, ground, one half teaspoon

Cumin, ground, one half teaspoon

Quorn Grounds, one bag*

Olive oil, one tablespoon

<u>Instructions</u>

Add the Quorn to the olive oil in a large skillet along with the salt, pepper, paprika, and cumin. Fry this for ten minutes. While the Quorn is frying mix the salad dressing and the salad greens in a large serving bowl. Pour the Quorn taco grounds on top of the greens, add on the nutritional yeast, and the guacamole and serve.

*To make this vegan substitute two cups of shredded jackfruit for the Quorn shreds and prepare the recipe the same way.

Taco Salad Dressing

If you do not like the cilantro that is in this recipe, just substitute it for parsley. While this dressing is meant for taco salad, it is also good on roasted veggies or as a meat marinade. It remains fresh in your refrigerator for two weeks.

<u>Ingredients</u>

Cumin, ground, one half teaspoon

Paprika, ground, one fourth teaspoon

Sea salt, one teaspoon

Dijon mustard, one teaspoon

Green onions, minced, one fourth cup

Cilantro, minced, one fourth cup

Garlic, minced, one tablespoon

Lime juice, one tablespoon

Red wine vinegar, one fourth cup

Olive oil, one half cup

<u>Instructions</u>

Blend all of these ingredients in a blender and then store the recipe in your refrigerator in a glass jar that has a tight-fitting lid.

Basic Guacamole

This recipe is free of lectins because it has no tomatoes added to it. It does have plenty of ingredients that make it tasty and healthy. You can keep this fresh in the refrigerator for up to five days. Before you refrigerate the guacamole, pour a thin layer of avocado oil or olive oil over it to keep the top fresh. When serving, you can either pour the oil off or blend it in.

Shopping list

cilantro or parsley, red onion, hot sauce, avocado

Ingredients

Lime juice, two tablespoons

Sea salt, one teaspoon

Black pepper, one teaspoon

Cumin, ground, one teaspoon

Cilantro or parsley, minced, one fourth cup

Red onion, one half minced

Garlic, minced, one tablespoon

Hot sauce, one teaspoon

Avocados, two ripe, pits removed, and cut in half.

Instructions

Mash the avocado pulp in a large bowl with a fork or a potato masher. Blend in all of the remaining ingredients and stir everything together well.

Chapter 6
Breakfast Recipes

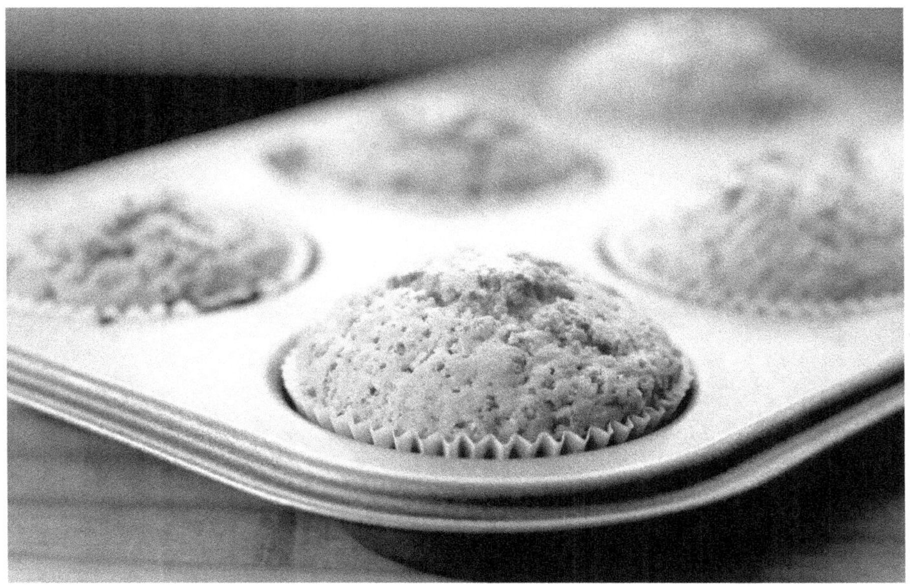

These recipes are suitable for Phase Two and/or Phase Three.

Almond Muffins

Makes twelve muffins

<u>Shopping list</u>

bittersweet chocolate, pastured eggs, shredded coconut, coconut flour, almond meal

<u>Ingredients</u>

Almonds, skinless slivered blanched, one half cup

Bittersweet chocolate, seventy-two percent cacaos or higher, chopped, one half cup

Almond extract, one teaspoon

Vanilla extract, one teaspoon

Coconut oil, melted, four tablespoons

Coconut milk, unsweetened, one third cup

Pastured eggs (or comparable egg substitute for vegan), three

Baking soda, one teaspoon

Erythritol, six tablespoons

Shredded coconut, unsweetened, one half cup

Coconut flour, one half cup

Almond meal, one cup

Instructions

Heat the oven to 375. Put muffin papers into a twelve cup muffin pan and set it off to the side. Use a large mixing bowl to mix together the baking soda, Erythritol, coconut, coconut flour, and almond meal until they are well blended. Set this bowl off to the side. In another mixing bowl, cream together the almond and vanilla extracts, coconut oil, coconut milk, and the eggs or egg replacer. Blend all of the ingredients together in one bowl and fold them over until they are well mixed. Combine the chocolate into the batter, and evenly divide the batter among the twelve paper muffin cups. Top each raw muffin with the slivered almonds and then bake the muffins for twenty-five minutes.

Green Egg Muffins

Makes twelve muffins

<u>Shopping list</u>

nutritional yeast, baby spinach, kale, yellow onion, pastured eggs

<u>Ingredients</u>

Nutritional yeast, one half cup

Coconut milk, unsweetened, one cup

Nutmeg, ground, one half teaspoon

Black pepper, one half teaspoon

Sea salt, one teaspoon

Baby spinach, two cups

Kale, shredded with stems removed, two cups

Yellow onion, one minced

Olive oil, two tablespoons

Pastured eggs, three

<u>Instructions</u>

Heat the oven to 375.

Line twelve cups of a muffin pan with muffin papers and set the pan to the side. Beat the eggs until they are smooth. Fry the onions for three minutes in the olive oil. Stir in the nutmeg, salt, pepper, spinach, and kale until they are well mixed and fry this for five minutes more. Carefully put the cooked greens in a blender with the coconut milk and puree until they are creamy and smooth. Then blend in the nutritional yeast and the eggs and divide the mixture evenly among the twelve muffin cups. Bake the muffins for twenty minutes.

Baked Avocado Cups with Pesto

Makes four cups

<u>**Shopping list**</u>

pesto, basil pesto, pastured eggs, prosciutto, avocados

Ingredients

Pesto of your choice to serve

Lemon juice, one tablespoon

Basil pesto, one fourth cup

Pastured eggs, four

Prosciutto, four slices

Avocados, two

Instructions

Heat the oven to 400. Slice the avocados in half around the middle and take out the pit and discard it. Scoop out some of the extra pulp of the avocado until it looks like a bowl. Line each bowl with one slice of the prosciutto. Set each avocado half into the cup of a muffin pan with the center hole facing up. Break one egg into each of the avocado holes and then put one teaspoon of the basil pesto on top of each egg and drizzle with the lemon juice. Bake the avocados for fifteen minutes. Serve them with the pesto dressing for serving.

Seasonal Fruit Salsa

Makes two cups

<u>**Shopping list**</u>

seasonal fruit, red onion, avocado

<u>**Ingredients**</u>

Seasonal fruit, diced, one cup

Cilantro, minced, one fourth cup

Lime juice, four tablespoons

Red wine vinegar, one tablespoon

Olive oil, one fourth cup

Sea salt, one teaspoon

Garlic, minced, two tablespoons

Hot sauce, one half teaspoon

Red onion, one minced

Avocado, one diced

<u>**Instructions**</u>

Toss together in a mixing bowl the salt, garlic, hot sauce, onion, avocado, cilantro, and the diced seasonal fruit until everything is well mixed. In a smaller bowl, blend together the lime juice, vinegar, and olive oil. Pour the olive oil mixture over the fruit mixture and toss this together well.

Avocado Cloud Bread

Makes twelve buns

avocado, pastured eggs

Ingredients

Sesame seeds, one teaspoon

Sea salt, one fourth teaspoon

Avocado, ripe, one half mashed

Cream of tartar, one fourth teaspoon

Pastured eggs, three separated

Instructions

Heat the oven to 300. Lay a baking mat made of silicone or parchment paper on a baking sheet and set it to the side. Cream together the cream of tartar and the egg whites for about four minutes until they make stiff peaks. In another bowl, blend together the salt, avocado, and the egg yolks. Put one-fourth of the egg white mixture into the mixture of egg yolk to make it lighter, and then put the egg yolk mixture into the egg white mixture and fold carefully to mix. Place a quarter of a cup size of batter onto the baking pan, so they are about two inches apart. Then sprinkle them with the sesame seeds and bake them for thirty minutes.

Carrot Cake Muffins

Makes twelve muffins

Shopping list

walnuts, carrots, pastured eggs, coconut flour, almond flour

Ingredients

Walnuts, chopped, one fourth cup

Carrots, two large grated finely

Vanilla extract, two teaspoons

Erythritol, one third cup

Coconut milk, unsweetened, two-thirds cup

Avocado oil, one third cup

Pastured eggs, two

Nutmeg, ground, one half teaspoon

Ginger, ground, one half teaspoon

Cinnamon, ground, two teaspoons

Sea salt, one eighth teaspoon

Baking soda, one half teaspoon

Coconut flour, two tablespoons

Almond flour, blanched, one and one fourth cups

Instructions

Heat the oven to 350. Line a twelve cup muffin pan with paper liners and set it to the side. Use a large mixing bowl to blend together the nutmeg, ginger, cinnamon, salt, baking soda, coconut flour, and the almond flour. Mix together in a separate smaller bowl the vanilla extract, Erythritol, coconut milk, avocado oil, and the eggs. Pour all of the ingredients together in one bowl and blend them together gently but well. Then stir in the chopped walnuts and the grated carrot. Divide the batter into twelve equal portions in the muffin pan and then bake them for eighteen minutes.

Plantain Pancakes

Serves four, two pancakes per person

<u>Shopping list</u>

pastured eggs, green plantains

<u>Ingredients</u>

Baking soda, one half teaspoon

Sea Salt, one eighth teaspoon

Erythritol, one fourth cup

Coconut oil, four tablespoons divided

Vanilla extract, two teaspoons

Pastured eggs, four

Green plantains, two large peeled and cut into chunks

<u>Instructions</u>

Mash or puree the pieces of plantain. Blend the eggs into the plantain to make a creamy batter. Then stir in the Erythritol, baking soda, salt, vanilla extract, and three tablespoons of the coconut oil. Beat this until it is well blended. Put the last tablespoon of coconut oil into a large skillet and pour one-half cup of the batter for each pancake you are cooking. Cook each pancake for five minutes on each side.

Orange Cranberry Muffins

Makes six muffins

<u>**Shopping list**</u>

dried cranberries, orange juice, pastured eggs, coconut flour

<u>**Ingredients**</u>

Cranberries, unsweetened and dried

Orange juice, one tablespoon

Pastured eggs, three

Xylitol, one fourth cup

Coconut oil, melted, one fourth cup

Baking soda, one fourth teaspoon

Sea salt, one fourth teaspoon

Coconut flour, one fourth cup

<u>**Instructions**</u>

Heat the oven to 350. Place paper cups in six cups of a six-cup muffin pan. Blend together well the xylitol, orange juice, eggs, baking soda, salt, and the coconut flour until all of the ingredients are well mixed. Gently stir in the cranberries and then divide the batter evenly among the six muffin cups. Bake the muffins for twenty minutes.

Cheesy Cauliflower Cups

Makes twelve cups

<u>**Shopping list**</u>

prosciutto, pastured eggs, spinach, Parmigiano-Reggiano cheese, riced cauliflower

Ingredients

Prosciutto, six slices cut into bits

Pastured eggs, four

Fresh spinach, chopped, one cup

Grated Parmigiano-Reggiano cheese, one cup

Cauliflower rice, thawed from frozen, five cups

Instructions

Heat the oven to 375. Blend together well the eggs, spinach, cauliflower rice, and one-half cup of the cheese in a large mixing bowl. Place muffin papers into a twelve cup muffin pan. Divide this mixture evenly among the muffin cups, then sprinkle on top the prosciutto and the remainder of the cheese. Bake these for fifteen minutes.

Spinach Cheese and Egg Breakfast Burrito

Makes four burritos

Shopping list

goat cheese, pastured eggs, spinach

Ingredients

Cassava flour tortillas, eight

Goat cheese, crumbled, four ounces

Pastured eggs, six-well beaten

Sea salt, one half teaspoon

Black pepper, one teaspoon

Garlic, minced, two tablespoons

Spinach, chopped, one quarter cup

Olive oil, two tablespoons

Instructions

Fry the salt, pepper, garlic, and the spinach for five minutes in the olive oil. Pour the beaten eggs slowly on top of the spinach mixture in the skillet and let them sit for three minutes, then scramble them until they are cooked the way that you like them. Spread the crumbled goat cheese on top of the eggs evenly and let it melt. While the cheese is melting, heat the tortillas in the microwave, then fill them evenly with the mix and serve.

Cassava Flour Tortillas

Shopping list

cassava flour, A2 protein butter

Ingredients

Cassava flour, one and one half cups

Warm water, one cup

Butter, A2 protein, one-quarter cup melted

<u>Instructions</u>

Blend the warm water and the butter together and then stir in the flour, working the dough with your hands until you have formed a soft dough ball. Then divide the dough ball into two-ounce portions. Put one of the portions between two pieces of parchment paper and roll it out to the thinness of a tortilla. Set a large skillet on a medium-high heat without using any grease or oil in the skillet, leave it dry. Gently peel both pieces of parchment paper off the rolled out tortilla and then lays it in the hot skillet. Let the tortilla cook for one to two minutes, no longer, and then use a large turner to flip the tortilla over and cook it for two minutes on the other side. Put the cooked tortillas in a two hundred degrees oven covered by a damp, clean dishtowel to make them moist and pliable.

Chapter 7
Lunch Recipes

These recipes are suitable for Phase Two and/or Phase Three.

Chicken Salad

Makes four servings

<u>Shopping list</u>

avocado, parsley, dill, jicama, celery, yellow onion, pasture-raised chicken

<u>Ingredients</u>

Sea salt, one teaspoon

Dijon mustard, one tablespoon

Rice wine vinegar, one tablespoon

Lemon juice, two tablespoons

Avocado oil, two tablespoons

Avocado, two

Parsley, minced, one tablespoon

Dill, minced, one tablespoon

Jicama, peeled and diced, one cup

Celery, minced, four ribs

Yellow onion, minced, one

Pasture-raised chicken, cooked and chopped, light or dark, two cups

<u>Instructions</u>

Toss together in a large bowl the parsley, dill, jicama, celery, onion, and the chicken until they are well mixed. Mash the pulp of the avocado and then cream it together with the sea salt, mustard, vinegar, lemon juice, and the avocado oil until it is creamy and smooth, adding a few drops of water if needed. Pour the dressing into the bowl of chicken mixture and fold all of the ingredients together until they are well mixed. Serve this with the Avocado Cloud Bread or on top of a bed of leafy greens.

Sesame Noodle Salad

Makes four servings

Shopping list

green onions, fresh mint, green onions, tahini, coconut aminos, yellow onion, broccoli, purple cabbage, shirataki noodles

Ingredients

Sesame seeds, for garnish, one fourth cup

Ginger, fresh, minced finely, two tablespoons

Green onions, minced finely, two

Mint, minced finely, one fourth cup

Monk fruit sweetener, one teaspoon

Lemon juice, two tablespoons

Garlic, minced, three tablespoons

Tahini, two tablespoons

Sesame oil, two tablespoons

Rice wine vinegar, two tablespoons

Coconut aminos, one fourth cup

Yellow onion, one sliced thinly

Broccoli, shredded, one cup

Purple cabbage, shredded, one half head

Shirataki noodles, two cups

Instructions

Blend well together in a large bowl the onion, broccoli, cabbage, and the shirataki noodles.

Then in a different bowl, mix together the sweetener, lemon juice, garlic, tahini, sesame oil,

rice vinegar, and the coconut aminos until all of the ingredients are well blended. Then stir

the ginger, green onion, and mint into the dressing and pour it over the noodles and toss

them well together. Serve the salad with the sesame seeds for garnish.

Millet Bowl

Makes one bowl

Shopping list

tahini, fresh herbs, avocado, asparagus, red onion, shrimp, millet, kale, sweet potato, shallot

Ingredients

Lemon juice, two tablespoons

Tahini, one teaspoon

Sesame seeds, one tablespoon

Minced fresh herbs, your choice, one fourth cup

Avocado, one-fourth of one

Asparagus, three spears

Red onion, minced, one fourth cup

Shrimp, wild-caught, one-half cup cooked

Millet, cooked, one cup

Kale, sliced finely, one cup

Sea salt, one half teaspoon

Sage, dried, one teaspoon

Sweet potato, minced, one half cup

Shallot, one minced

Olive oil, one tablespoon

Instructions

Fry the sweet potato, sea salt, sage, and shallot in the hot olive oil for three minutes. Add in the kale and fry it until the kale wilts, stirring often. Heat up the millet and put it in the bottom of a bowl, then put the sweet potato and kale mixture on top. Lay the shrimp, avocado, onion, and asparagus on top of this and garnish with the sesame seeds and the minced fresh herbs. Stir the lemon juice into the tahini and use this as a dressing for the bowl.

Collard Wrapped Burritos

Makes two burritos

<u>Shopping list</u>

coconut yogurt, rice cauliflower, Quorn grounds, collard greens

<u>Ingredients</u>

Coconut yogurt, one fourth cup

Guacamole, one fourth cup

Seasonal Fruit Salsa, one fourth cup

Cauliflower Rice, one half cup

Sea salt, one half teaspoon

Black pepper, one half teaspoon

Paprika, ground, one half teaspoon

Cumin, ground, one half teaspoon

Olive oil, one tablespoon

Quorn grounds, one bag*

Collard greens leaves, four large

Instructions

Chop the stems off the collard leaves, so they are no longer than the leaf itself, and then use a vegetable peeler to trim the rib until it is very thin. Simmer the leaves in boiling water for three minutes and then set them to the side. Fry the Quorn in the olive oil along with the salt, pepper, paprika, and cumin for five minutes. Warm the Cauliflower Rice in the microwave for two minutes, and then stir well. Lay down two of the collard leaves, letting them overlap about an inch. Spread half of the Cauliflower Rice on the leaves carefully, and then add on the Quorn mixture, salsa, and the guacamole. Sprinkle all of this with half of the yogurt, and then carefully roll the leaves into a burrito shape. Repeat with the other two leaves and the rest of the ingredients.

To make these vegan substitute two cups of shredded jackfruit for the Quorn.

Broccoli Pesto Noodles

Makes two servings

Shopping list

basil pesto, shirataki noodles, broccoli florets

Ingredients

Basil pesto, two tablespoons

Shirataki noodles, two cups

Broccoli florets, one cup

Olive oil, two tablespoons

<u>**Instructions**</u>

Heat the noodles in boiling water for five minutes. While the noodles are boiling, fry the broccoli in the olive oil for three minutes, then drain the noodles and add then in, cooking for five more minutes. Pour this mixture into a bowl and blend in the basil pesto and then serve.*Garlic Kale Sweet Potato*

Serves one

<u>**Shopping list**</u>

kale, sweet potato

<u>**Ingredients**</u>

Sea salt, one half teaspoon

Garlic, minced, one tablespoon

Kale, sliced, one cup

Olive oil, two tablespoons

Sweet potato, one six to eight-ounce size

<u>**Instructions**</u>

Heat the oven to 375. Wash and dry the sweet potato and then poke eight to ten holes in the skin with a fork to let the steam release. Bake the sweet potato for thirty to forty minutes or until it is soft. When the sweet potato is almost finished baking, fry the kale, garlic, and the sea salt in the hot olive oil for five minutes. Slice the sweet potato in half and then top the halves with the kale mixture and serve.

Portobello Mushroom Pizza

Serves two

Shopping list

buffalo mozzarella, prosciutto, basil pesto, Portobello mushrooms

Ingredients

Buffalo mozzarella, one ball sliced into one half-inch thick slices

Italian prosciutto, two slices

Basil pesto, six tablespoons

Olive oil, three tablespoons

Portobello mushrooms, two large with the stems removed

Instructions

Spread olive oil on the mushroom caps and grill them in a large skillet over a high heat, cap side up, for five minutes or until the caps begin to brown slightly. Turn the caps over and grill them for another five minutes. Into each of the mushroom caps, divide the basil pesto, and then lie on one slice of the prosciutto and cover with the sliced cheese. Leave the caps in the skillet until the cheese begins to melt and then serve.

Omelet and Salad

Serves one

Shopping list

arugula, pastured eggs

Ingredients

Sea salt, one half teaspoon

Balsamic vinegar, one tablespoon

Arugula, two cups

Olive oil, two tablespoons

Pastured eggs, three

Instructions

Blend together the balsamic vinegar with one tablespoon of the olive oil and set this to the side. Beat the eggs well together and stir in the sea salt. Pour the eggs into the rest of the olive oil in a large skillet and let the eggs cook, undisturbed, for four to five minutes, until the outside third of the eggs begins to look set. Then fold one half of the omelet carefully over the other half and cook for two more minutes on each side. Toss the olive oil and vinegar dressing that you made with the arugula and serve it with the omelet.

Bok Choy with Shrimp

Serves two

<u>Shopping list</u>

bok choy, wild-caught shrimp

<u>Ingredients</u>

Bok choy, sliced, three cups

Garlic, minced, three tablespoons

Ginger, freshly minced, one tablespoon

Sesame oil, one tablespoon

Wild-caught shrimp, six ounces

<u>Instructions</u>

Fry the garlic, ginger, and the shrimp in the hot sesame oil for five minutes. The shrimp will begin to turn pink. Mix in the bok choy and blend this well, then fry for another five minutes until the shrimp is fully cooked, and the bok choy is wilted, stirring occasionally.

Purple Root Vegetables Latkes

Makes eight to ten

Shopping list

pastured eggs, cassava flour, scallions, red onion, beet, parsnips, carrots, coconut yogurt

Ingredients

Olive oil, one-fourth cup divided

Black pepper, one teaspoon

Sea salt, one half teaspoon

Pastured eggs, two

Cassava flour, one half cup

Scallions, three sliced thinly

Red onion, peeled and diced finely, one fourth

Beet, one, peeled and shredded

Parsnips, three, peeled and shredded

Carrots, four, peeled and shredded

Coconut yogurt, one cup

Instructions

Heat the oven to 300. Mix together in a medium-sized bowl the grated carrots, parsnips, and beets along with the red onion. Blend in the salt, pepper, eggs, flour, and the scallions and mix this all together very well. Measure out a one-third cup of the mix and fry these in the hot oil for five minutes on each side on a medium heat, letting them drain briefly on a paper towel when they are finished cooking. Serve the latkes with the coconut yogurt for dipping.

Veggie Curry with Sweet Potato Noodles

Serves two

Shopping list

fresh parsley, sweet potato, onion, broccoli florets, carrot

Ingredients

SWEET POTATO NOODLES

Parsley, chopped for garnish, four tablespoons

Sweet potato, one large peeled and cut in spirals

Sea salt, one half teaspoon

Coconut oil, one half tablespoon

CURRY

Sea salt, one half teaspoon

Coconut milk, one can

Yellow curry powder, one tablespoon

Ginger, dried, one half teaspoon

Onion, minced, one third cup

Broccoli florets, one cup

Carrot, one large peeled and cut into spirals

Coconut oil, one half tablespoon

<u>Instructions</u>

Put the coconut oil in a pan over medium-high heat and stir in the carrot and cook for three minutes. Lower the heat and stir in the ginger, onion, and broccoli and mix well, then cook this mixture for five minutes. Stir in the coconut milk and the yellow curry powder and cook for one minute more and then boil it. Then let the mixture simmer for fifteen minutes, stirring the mix occasionally until the sauce becomes thick. While you are cooking the sauce cook the spiral sweet potatoes in the coconut oil for ten minutes. Stir in the salt as they cook. Pour the cooked sauce on top of the cooked noodles to serve and garnish them with the chopped parsley.

Baked Artichoke Hearts

Serves two

Shopping list

cassava flour, artichoke hearts

Ingredients

Black pepper, one fourth teaspoon

Sea salt, one half teaspoon

Cassava flour, one cup

Artichoke hearts, ten

Cayenne pepper, one eighth teaspoon

Lemon juice, two tablespoons

Olive oil, four tablespoons

Instructions

Heat the oven to 400. Mix together the cayenne pepper, lemon juice, and three tablespoons

of the olive oil until they are well blended, then drop in the artichoke hearts and toss gently to coat them with this mixture. Use the last tablespoon of the olive oil to grease a baking sheet. Blend together the salt, pepper, and the flour in a bowl and drop in the artichoke hearts, mixing them well until they are well coated with the flour. Set the artichoke hearts on the oiled baking sheet and bake them for thirty minutes.

Romaine Lettuce Boats with Guacamole

Serves one

Shopping list

romaine lettuce, fresh cilantro, red onion, avocado

Ingredients

Romaine lettuce leaves, four washed and dried

Sea salt, one half teaspoon

Lemon juice, one tablespoon

Cilantro, chopped finely, one teaspoon

Red onion, chopped finely, one tablespoon

Avocado, one half of one

Instructions

Mash the pulp of the avocado with the red onion, sea salt, and the lemon juice.

Lay one romaine lettuce leaf on top of another and put half of the avocado mix on it, then garnish it with half of the cilantro. Roll the leaves up and enjoy.

Millet Cakes

Serves four

Shopping list

coconut flour, pastured eggs, mushrooms, fresh basil, carrots, red onion, vegetable broth, millet

Ingredients

Coconut flour, one tablespoon

Pastured eggs, one

Olive oil, two tablespoons

Italian seasoning, one half teaspoon

Garlic, minced, one tablespoon

Mushrooms, chopped finely, one cup

Basil, chopped finely, one fourth cup

Carrots, chopped finely, one fourth cup

Red onion, chopped finely, one fourth cup

Sea salt, one teaspoon

Vegetable broth, two cups

Millet, one half cup

Instructions

Put the millet into a dry pan over a high heat and toast it for five minutes, stirring it often to prevent burning. Then pour in the salt and the vegetable broth carefully and let it boil.

Then simmer the millet for fifteen minutes until all of the liquid is absorbed by the millet. Set it off to the side and let it stand for ten minutes before fluffing the millet with a fork.

Fry the veggies in one tablespoon of the olive oil for five minutes, stirring often. Then stir in the coconut four, beaten egg, and the millet and mix well, then remove this mixture from the heat and let it cool to room temperature. Then form the mixture into patties and fry them in the last tablespoon of the oil for five minutes on each side.

Broccoli Puffs

Makes twenty

Shopping list

nutritional yeast, hot sauce, fresh parsley, almond meal, cassava flour, yellow onion, pastured eggs, broccoli florets

Ingredients

Hot sauce or guacamole for dipping

Nutritional yeast, one fourth cup

Parsley, minced, one tablespoon

Sea salt, one teaspoon

Black pepper, one half teaspoon

Almond meal, one fourth cup

Cassava flour, one half cup

Garlic, minced, one tablespoon

Yellow onion, minced, one half of one

Pastured egg, one

Broccoli florets, two cups steamed

Spray olive oil

<u>**Instructions**</u>

Heat the oven to 400. Use the spray oil to grease a baking sheet. Chop the broccoli florets and mix them with the remainder of the ingredients until everything is well mixed together. Form the mixture into shapes that look like potato puffs using one tablespoon of the mixture for each puff. Bake the puffs for fifteen minutes.

Chapter 8
Dinner Recipes

These recipes are suitable for Phase Two and/or Phase Three.

Shrimp Risotto

Makes six servings

Shopping list

nutritional yeast, vegetables broth, riced cauliflower, asparagus, fresh parsley, shallots, wild-caught shrimp

Ingredients

Black pepper, one teaspoon

Sea salt, one half teaspoon

Lemon juice, two tablespoons

Nutritional yeast, one fourth cup

Vegetable broth, two cups

Cauliflower rice, two sixteen-ounce packages

Asparagus, cut into bite-sized chunks, two cups

Lemon zest, two tablespoons

Paprika, one half teaspoon

Sea salt, one half teaspoon

Parsley, fresh minced, one fourth cup

Garlic, minced, three tablespoons

Shallots, minced, four

Olive oil, one fourth cup

Wild-caught shrimp, peeled and deveined,

Coconut milk, unsweetened, one thirteen to fourteen ounce can

Instructions

Simmer the coconut milk and the shrimp in a pot over medium heat. In a larger pan, fry the garlic and shallots in the olive oil for five minutes, stirring occasionally. Drain the shrimp out of the coconut milk and put it into this mixture along with the paprika, salt, pepper, and parsley with half of the lemon zest, saving the coconut milk. Cook all of this mixture for five minutes, stirring often. Then add in the asparagus and cook for five more minutes. Then add the cauliflower rice and cook this for ten or fifteen more minutes, or until all of the liquid is gone. Then stir in the rest of the lemon zest with the lemon juice, nutritional yeast, broth, and the reserved coconut milk and cook this on simmer for ten minutes or until the sauce has thickened.

Veggie Noodle Bake

Makes eight servings

Shopping list

almond meal, nutritional yeast, meat or seafood per recipe, zucchini noodles, kale or baby spinach, Brussels sprouts, yellow onion, asparagus

Ingredients

Nutritional yeast, one half cup

Almond meal, one half cup

Allowed meat or seafood of choice, two cups

Vegan Nut Cheese sauce, one cup

Zucchini noodles, four cups, cooked

Paprika, ground, one half teaspoon

Black pepper, one half teaspoon

Sea salt, one teaspoon

Sage, dried, one tablespoon

Thyme, dried, one tablespoon

Garlic, minced, two tablespoons

Kale or baby spinach, stems removed, three cups

Brussels sprouts,

Asparagus, one bunch, chopped into bite-sized pieces

Yellow onion, one large chopped

Olive oil, one tablespoon

Olive oil spray

Instructions

Heat the oven to 375. Use the olive oil spray to spray a thirteen by nine-inch baking dish and set it to the side. Fry the Brussels sprouts, asparagus, and onion in the hot olive oil for seven to nine minutes. Mix in the paprika, pepper, salt, sage, thyme, garlic, and the greens and cook this, stirring occasionally, until the greens have wilted. Drain the excess liquid off of this mixture. Mix the cheese sauce with the zucchini noodles in a large bowl and then gently mix the strained veggies into the mix in the bowl. Put all of this mixture into the baking dish and then sprinkle the nutritional yeast and the almond meal on top and then bake the casserole for forty minutes.

Vegan Nut Cheese Sauce

Makes two cups

Shopping list

nutritional yeast, raw macadamia nuts, one lemon

Ingredients

Sea salt, one teaspoon

Onion powder, one teaspoon

Black pepper, one teaspoon

Garlic powder, one teaspoon

Paprika, ground, one teaspoon

Nutritional yeast, one fourth cup

Lemon juice, two tablespoons

Lemon zest, two tablespoons

Macadamia nuts, raw, two cups soaked in water for four hours

Instructions

Drain the soaking water off the macadamia nuts and throw the water away. Blend the macadamia nuts with the salt, spices, nutritional yeast, lemon juice, and lemon zest until all of the ingredients are creamy and smooth. If needed, add a few drops of water at a time to maintain a creamy consistency.

Chicken and Veggies

Makes four servings

Shopping list

one lemon, asparagus, cauliflower florets, broccoli florets, four pasture-raised chicken thighs

Ingredients

Lemon, one, sliced thinly

Asparagus, chopped into bite-sized pieces, one cup

Cauliflower florets, one cup

Broccoli florets, two cups

Garlic, minced, two tablespoons

Rosemary, dried, one eighth cup

Avocado oil, one fourth cup

Sea salt, one and one-half teaspoons divided

Chicken, pasture-raised, four chicken thighs

Instructions

Heat the oven to 425. Season the chicken with one-half teaspoon of the sea salt. Use a large-sized bowl to blend together the garlic, rosemary, avocado oil, and the rest of the salt. Then add in the sliced lemon, shallots, asparagus, cauliflower, and broccoli and toss them gently but thoroughly to coat all of the pieces well. Spread the mixture of veggies out onto a baking sheet around the pieces of chicken and bake the food for forty minutes.

Beef and Mushrooms

Makes four servings

Shopping list

one from the first three ingredients, beef broth, one lemon, mushrooms, celery, onion, cassava flour, grass-fed sirloin

<u>Ingredients</u>

Cauliflower Rice, Cooked Millet, or Spinach Risotto for serving, four cups

Red wine vinegar, one tablespoon

Beef broth, three-fourths cup

Balsamic vinegar, one half cup

Lemon zest, one tablespoon

Sea salt, one teaspoon

Seafood Spice Rub, one tablespoon

Rosemary, fresh, minced, one tablespoon

Thyme, dried, one tablespoon

Mushrooms, trimmed and sliced, one cup

Garlic, minced, two tablespoons

Celery, minced, two ribs

Onion, one minced

Olive oil, one fourth cup

Cassava flour, one tablespoon

Grass-fed sirloin, one-half pound cubed

<u>Instructions</u>

Coat the sirloin cubes with the cassava flour and fry it in the hot olive oil for five minutes, stirring frequently. Mix in the mushrooms, garlic, celery, and onion and fry this for six more minutes. Blend in the lemon zest, sea salt, spice rub, rosemary, and thyme and cook for an additional two minutes. Pour in the broth and both kinds of vinegar and stir the skillet quickly, scraping the bottom of the skillet to deglaze the skillet. Simmer this mixture for forty-five minutes until the beef is tender and the sauce has become thick. Serve over the cauliflower rice, cooked millet, or the spinach risotto.

Creamy Mac and Cheese

Makes four servings

Shopping list

nutritional yeast, almond milk, one head of cauliflower, red lentil pasta

Ingredients

Olive oil and chopped parsley for serving

Italian seasoning, one half teaspoon

Nutritional yeast, two tablespoons

Garlic, minced, two tablespoons

Almond milk, plain, one cup

Cauliflower, one head cut into florets

Sea salt, one half teaspoon

Black pepper, one teaspoon

Red lentil pasta, one eight-ounce box cooked

Instructions

Mix the garlic, milk, and cauliflower in a pot and cook this for fifteen minutes. Then stir in the pepper, salt, Italian seasoning, nutritional yeast, and a quarter cup of water and then blend this mixture until it is creamy and smooth. Then pour this sauce over the pasta and toss gently to mix completely. Serve the mac and cheese with the olive oil and parsley for a garnish.

Flaky Fried Fish

Makes four servings

Shopping list

wild-caught mahi-mahi, fresh basil, asparagus

Ingredients

Mahi-mahi, wild-caught, four four-ounce pieces

Olive oil, one fourth cup

Garlic, minced, two tablespoons

Basil, fresh, one fourth cup

Black pepper, one teaspoon

Sea salt, one half cup

Olive oil, two tablespoons to brush on the fish

Asparagus, two pounds thin stalks

Instructions

Steam the asparagus for six to ten minutes until done. While they are steaming, brush the olive oil on the fish and season the fillets with the salt and pepper. Fry these in a hot skillet for five minutes on each side. In a small bowl, blend together the olive oil, lemon zest, garlic, and basil and use this as a sauce to spoon over the fish and asparagus.

Chicken Arugula Salad with Lemon Vinaigrette

Serves one

Shopping list

mushrooms, arugula, four ounces of pasture-raised chicken breast

Ingredients

Mushrooms, canned, drained and rinsed, one small can

Arugula, one and one half cups

Sea salt, one-half teaspoon and one fourth teaspoon

Lemon juice, one tablespoon

Olive oil, two tablespoons

Chicken breast, pasture-raised, four ounces cut into strips one half-inch thick*

Avocado oil, one tablespoon

Instructions

Fry the chicken strips in the avocado oil and sprinkle them with the lemon juice and the one-half teaspoon of salt. Cook the strips of chicken for three minutes on each side. Take the chicken from the skillet and set it to the side. Mix together to make the dressing for the salad the olive oil, lemon juice, and the one-fourth cup teaspoon of salt. Mix the mushrooms with the arugula and serve with the chicken and dressing.

Make this recipe vegan by replacing the chicken with hemp tofu or grain-free tempeh.

Chicken Seaweed Wraps

Serves one

Shopping list

fresh cilantro, large green olives, Nori seaweed, arugula, avocado, four ounces of pasture-raised chicken breast

Ingredients

DIPPING SAUCE

Sea salt, one fourth cup

Lemon juice, two tablespoons

Olive oil, one fourth cup

Cilantro, chopped, two cups

WRAP FILLING

Green olives, four pitted and sliced

Nori seaweed, one-sheet

Arugula, one cup

Avocado, diced, one half cup

Sea salt, one fourth teaspoon

Lemon juice, two tablespoons

Pasture-raised chicken breast, four ounces sliced into strips*

Avocado oil, one tablespoon

Instructions

DIPPING SAUCE

Blend together the cilantro, olive oil, lemon juice, and the sea salt in a blender and mix it until it is creamy and smooth. Set this off to the side.

FILLING MIX

Fry the chicken strips in the avocado oil and fry them for four minutes on each side, seasoning them with the salt and the lemon juice. Add the avocado in and cook for another four minutes.

Lay out a sheet of seaweed and cover it with the arugula. Cover the arugula with the olives, avocado, and the chicken. Roll the sheet of seaweed up tightly and serve it with the dipping sauce.

Make this vegan by substituting the chicken with hemp tofu or grain-free tempeh.

Cabbage Steaks with Lemony Kale and Brussels Sprouts

Serves one

<u>Shopping list</u>

kale, Brussels sprouts, red onion, red cabbage

<u>Ingredients</u>

Lemon juice, one tablespoon

Kale, chopped, one and one half cups

Brussels sprouts, thinly sliced, one cup

Red onion, one half of one, thinly sliced

Sea salt, one fourth teaspoon

Red cabbage, one slice that is one inch thick

Avocado oil, four tablespoons

Instructions

Sear the slice of cabbage in one tablespoon of the avocado oil for five minutes on each side.

Put the slice of cabbage on a plate and set it to the side. Add two tablespoons of the avocado

oil to the skillet and fry the Brussels sprout and onions for four minutes, stirring frequently.

Mix in the last remaining tablespoon of avocado oil with the lemon juice and the kale and fry

this for three more minutes. Sprinkle the salt on this mixture and then serve it on top of the

cabbage steak.

Roasted Broccoli with Rice and Onions

Serves one

Shopping list

 red onion, broccoli florets, cauliflower head

Ingredients

CURRIED ONIONS

Sea salt, one fourth teaspoon

Red onion, thinly sliced, one half of one

Avocado oil, one half teaspoon

BROCCOLI

Sea salt, one fourth teaspoon

Avocado oil, two tablespoons

Broccoli florets, one and one half cups

CAULIFLOWER RICE

Sea salt, one fourth teaspoon

Curry powder, one fourth teaspoon

Lemon juice, one tablespoon

Avocado oil, one tablespoon

Cauliflower, one half of one medium-sized head, riced

Instructions

Heat the oven to 325. Fry the riced cauliflower in one tablespoon of the avocado oil with the salt, curry powder, and lemon juice for five minutes. Remove the riced cauliflower from the skillet and put it in a covered bowl to keep warm and set it off to the side. Set the broccoli florets into a baking dish with one tablespoon of the avocado oil and toss to coat them thoroughly and sprinkle them with the sea salt. Roast these in the oven for fifteen minutes. Fry the slices of onion in the avocado oil with the sea salt for five minutes. To serve, put the riced cauliflower on a plate and place the fried onions and the roasted broccoli on top.

Swedish Meatballs

Serves four

<u>Shopping list</u>

coconut cream, fish sauce, coconut aminos, vegetable broth, white mushrooms, white onion, almond flour, zucchini noodles, pastured eggs, grass-fed ground beef

<u>Ingredients</u>

<u>SAUCE</u>

Sea salt, one half teaspoon

Black pepper, one teaspoon

Parsley, dried, two tablespoons

Coconut cream, three-fourths cup

Garlic powder, one teaspoon

Balsamic vinegar, one teaspoon

Ground mustard, one fourth teaspoon

Fish sauce, one teaspoon

Coconut aminos, one half tablespoon

Vegetable broth, two cups

White mushrooms, four large sliced

White onion, sliced, one half cup

Coconut oil, one tablespoon

MEATBALLS

Black pepper, one fourth teaspoon

Sea salt, one teaspoon

Almond flour, three tablespoons

Parsley, dried, two tablespoons

Mustard powder, one fourth teaspoon

Onion powder, one teaspoon

White onion, minced, one fourth cup

White mushrooms, four large minced

Pasture-raised egg, one

Grass-fed ground beef, one pound

Zucchini noodles, two cups

<u>**Instructions**</u>

Heat the oven to 425. Fit a sheet of aluminum foil to the top of a baking sheet. Blend together in a medium-sized bowl the almond flour, parsley, salt, pepper, mustard powder, onion powder, egg, mushroom, minced onion, and the ground beef until all of the ingredients are well mixed. Portion the mix out into small meatballs and roll them up. Put the meatballs on the baking sheet and bake the meatballs for twenty minutes. Make the meatball sauce while the meatballs are in the oven. Fry the mushrooms and onions in the hot oil for four minutes and then pour in the vegetable broth to deglaze the skillet. Blend in the fish sauce, balsamic vinegar, coconut aminos, salt, pepper, ground mustard, and garlic powder and mix well. Let this cook for five minutes. Add in the baked meatballs and simmer this for ten minutes, stirring often, while the sauce thickens. Take off the skillet from the heat and mix in the coconut cream. Serve the mixture over the zucchini noodles.

Orange Chicken with Cranberry Sauce

Serves four

<u>**Shopping list**</u>

orange juice, one orange, fresh cranberries, Brussels sprouts, four pasture-raised boneless skinless chicken thighs

<u>**Ingredients**</u>

<u>**CRANBERRY SAUCE**</u>

Water, one fourth cup

Orange juice, two tablespoons

Orange zest, one tablespoon

Monk fruit sweetener, one tablespoon

Cranberries, fresh, one cup

BRUSSELS SPROUTS

Avocado oil, one tablespoon

Sea salt, one half teaspoon

Black pepper, one teaspoon

Brussels sprouts, one pound cut in half

CHICKEN

Orange juice, one tablespoon

Sea salt, one half teaspoon

Black pepper, one teaspoon

Poultry spice, one tablespoon

Boneless chicken thighs, pasture-raised, four

Instructions

Heat the oven to 375. Pat the chicken thighs dry. Mix in a bowl the orange juice, poultry spice, salt, and pepper and let the thighs marinate for one hour. Then cook the thighs in a baking dish in the hot oven for twenty minutes. While the chicken is baking, toss the Brussels sprouts with the avocado oil, salt, and pepper. Add the Brussels sprouts to the baking dish after twenty minutes and bake all of this for twenty minutes more. While it is baking, make the cranberry sauce by putting the rinsed cranberries into a pot over a medium-high heat with the water, orange juice, orange zest, and monk fruit sweetener. Cook this for twenty minutes. The sauce will thicken, and the cranberries will pop open. Serve the cranberry sauce with the chicken and Brussels sprouts.

Creamy Mushrooms and Chicken

Serves four

<u>Shopping list</u>

celery, onions, parsnips, carrots, fennel, arrowroot flour, chicken broth, fresh parsley, crimini mushrooms

<u>Ingredients</u>

<u>CHICKEN BROTH</u>

Sea salt, one teaspoon

Black peppercorns, one half teaspoon

Bay leaves, two

Celery, diced, one half cup

Onions, diced, one half cup

Parsnips, diced, one half cup

Carrots, diced, one half cup

Fennel, diced, one half cup

CREAMY MUSHROOM AND CHICKEN

Lemon juice, two tablespoons

Sea salt, one teaspoon

Black pepper, one teaspoon

Avocado oil, two tablespoons

Arrowroot flour, two tablespoons dissolved in cold water

Chicken broth, one cup

Coconut milk, one can

Parsley, fresh, one bunch washed, dried, and chopped

Thyme, dried, one fourth teaspoon

Garlic, minced, three tablespoons

Crimini mushrooms, twenty whole, washed, dried, and sliced

Instructions

Prepare the chicken broth by putting all of the ingredients for the broth into four cups of water and boil. Then let this broth simmer for thirty minutes. Then remove the chicken and set it off to the side. Take out the bay leaves and throw them away. Strain out the cooked veggies and set them in a bowl off to the side. Make the mushrooms by putting the avocado oil in a skillet over a medium heat and adding in the garlic and the mushrooms. Fry them for fifteen minutes, stirring occasionally. While the mushrooms are frying shred the chicken. Then put the shredded chicken in the skillet with one cup of the broth and the coconut milk and boil. Then let the mixture simmer for ten minutes, so the sauce will begin to get thick. Add the moistened arrowroot to the skillet and blend in well, then cook for five more minutes. Serve with the mixed veggie son the side and garnish with the chopped parsley.

Spinach Stuffed Chicken Breast

Serves four

Shopping list

 avocado mayonnaise, nutritional yeast, spinach, four pasture-raised chicken breasts

Ingredients

Avocado oil, two tablespoons

Sea salt, one half teaspoon

Black pepper, one teaspoon

Oregano, one teaspoon

Garlic powder, one fourth teaspoon

Paprika, ground, two teaspoons

Italian seasoning, two teaspoons

Avocado mayonnaise, three tablespoons

Nutritional yeast, one cup

Spinach, two bunches

Chicken breast, pasture-raised, four

<u>**Instructions**</u>

Heat the oven to 375. Wash the spinach and steam it for three minutes until it wilts, then drain it and chop it finely. Drop the spinach into a bowl with the nutritional yeast and the mayonnaise and blend well together. Cut a line in one side of each of the chicken breasts with a sharp knife, cutting about halfway through without cutting all the way through. Use the salt, pepper, and Italian seasoning to season inside of the chicken breasts and then stuff some of the spinach mixture inside of the chicken breasts. Use the oregano, paprika, and garlic powder to season the outside of the breasts and then bake them in the oven for forty minutes. Let the breasts rest for ten minutes before you serve them

Chapter 9
Smoothie Recipes

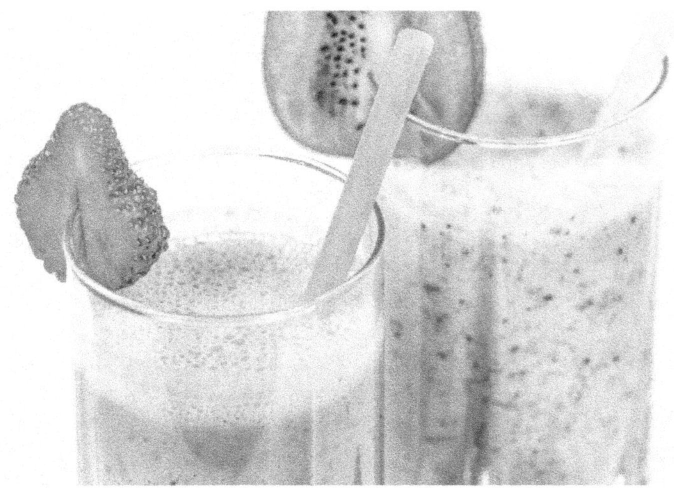

Smoothies are some of the best things for quenching hunger between meals or starting off your day. Mix all smoothie ingredients in the blender until they are creamy and smooth. Only make the fruit smoothies when that fruit is in season.

Purple Smoothie

<u>Shopping list</u>

frozen berries, purple sweet potato, baby spinach, coconut yogur*t*

Ingredients

Frozen berries, one cup

Purple sweet potato, baked and cooled, one fourth cup

Baby spinach, one cup

Coconut yogurt, one fourth cup

Almond milk, three-fourths cup

Carrot Smoothie

Shopping list

carrot juice, coconut yogurt, kale

Ingredients

Carrot juice, one cup

Coconut yogurt, one cup

Chocolate Smoothie

Shopping list

hemp seeds, avocado

Ingredients

Hemp seeds, one tablespoon

Cocoa powder, raw organic, two tablespoons

Stevia, four drops

Avocado, one half of one

Almond milk, unsweetened, two cups

Strawberry Smoothie

Shopping list

strawberries fresh or frozen, baby spinach

Ingredients

Strawberries, one cup

Baby spinach, one cup

Coconut yogurt, one cup

Cinnamon, one teaspoon

Raspberry Orange

Shopping list

 orange juice, frozen raspberries, coconut yogurt

Ingredients

Orange juice, one cup

Raspberries, frozen, one cup

Coconut yogurt, one half cup

Ice, one cup

Peach Smoothie

Shopping list

frozen peaches, coconut yogurt, avocado, fresh mint

Ingredients

Peaches, frozen, one cup

Coconut yogurt, one cup

Avocado, one half of one

Mint, chopped, one tablespoon

Kale, chopped, one cup

Ice, one cup

Zucchini Smoothie

Shopping list

frozen zucchini, almond milk, avocado

Ingredients

Zucchini, frozen, one cup

Almond milk, one half cup

Avocado, one half of one

Carrot Ginger Cumin Smoothie

Shopping list

almond milk, carrot juice

Ingredients

Almond milk, unsweetened, one cup

Lemon juice, one tablespoon

Carrot juice, one half cup

Cumin, ground, one teaspoon

Ginger, ground, one teaspoon

Ice, one cup

Blueberry Zucchini Smoothie

<u>Shopping list</u>

almond milk, zucchini, frozen blueberries

<u>Ingredients</u>

Ice, one cup

Almond milk, one half cup

Zucchini, chopped, one cup frozen

Blueberries, frozen, one cup

Beet Smoothie

<u>Shopping list</u>

 fresh beets, coconut yogurt, avocado

<u>Ingredients</u>

Beets, four peeled

Coconut yogurt, one cup

Avocado, one frozen

Chapter 10
Soup Recipes

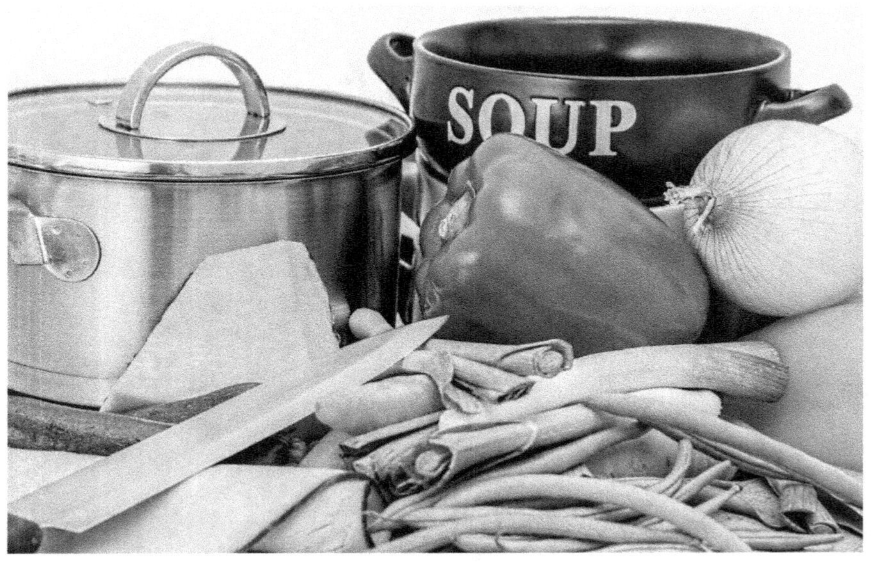

These recipes are suitable for Phase Two and/or Phase Three unless otherwise noted.

Garlicky Greens Soup

Makes six servings

Shopping list

vegetables broth, spinach, Swiss chard, celery, onion, nutritional yeast

Ingredients

Lemon juice, one tablespoon

Vegetable broth, six cups

Spinach, shredded, two cups

Swiss chard, shredded, two cups

Mustard powder, one half teaspoon

Black pepper, one teaspoon

Sea salt, one teaspoon

Paprika, ground, one teaspoon

Garlic powder, one teaspoon

Garlic, minced, three tablespoons

Celery, minced, two stalks

Onion, diced finely, one medium-sized

Olive oil, three tablespoons

Nutritional yeast for garnish

Instructions

Fry the garlic, celery, and onion in a large soup pot in the olive oil for five minutes, stirring occasionally. Mix in the mustard powder, salt, pepper, paprika, and the garlic powder and fry for two more minutes. Then add in the greens and cook them until they are wilted, about seven minutes. Pour in the lemon juice and the broth and let the soup simmer for twenty minutes. Garnish each bowl with nutritional yeast for serving if desired.

Lentil Chili (Phase Three Only)

Makes six servings

Shopping list

fresh cilantro, nutritional yeast, vegetables broth, fresh tomatoes, red or black dried lentils, jalapeno pepper, red bell pepper, celery, onion

Ingredients

Cilantro, minced, one cup for serving

Nutritional yeast for serving

Black pepper, one teaspoon

Sea salt, one teaspoon

Cloves, ground, one fourth teaspoon

Cinnamon, ground, one half teaspoon

Cumin, ground, one tablespoon

Chili powder, three tablespoons

Vegetable broth, five cups

Tomatoes, six large peeled with the seeds removed, chopped small

Lentils, red or black, three cups

Garlic, minced, three tablespoons

Jalapeno pepper, one peeled with the seeds removed and diced

Red bell pepper, one peeled with the seeds removed and diced

Celery, minced, three stalks

Onion, one large chopped

Olive oil, one fourth cup

Instructions

Fry the garlic, peppers, celery, and the onions in the hot olive oil for five minutes. Stir in the salt, pepper, cloves, cinnamon, cumin, chili powder, tomatoes, lentils, and the vegetable broth and blend the entire ingredients together well. Boil this chili and then let it simmer for thirty minutes. Serve the chili topped with minced cilantro or nutritional yeast as desired.

Sweet Potato Soup

Makes four servings

Shopping list

vegetables broth, fennel bulb, red onion, sweet potato, cauliflower head

Ingredient

Vegetable broth, four cups

Sea salt, one teaspoon

Black pepper, one teaspoon

Garlic, minced, two tablespoons

Ginger, ground, one tablespoon

Turmeric, ground, one teaspoon

Fennel bulb, one chopped

Red onion, one chopped

Sweet potato cubes, two cups

Cauliflower florets, two cups

Instructions

Boil all of the ingredients in a large pot over a high heat, and then simmer the soup for thirty minutes.

Leek Cauliflower Soup

Makes six servings

Shopping list

nutritional yeast, vegetable broth, cauliflower head, celery, leeks

Ingredients

Black pepper, one teaspoon

Sea salt, one teaspoon

Nutmeg, ground, one half teaspoon

Bay leaf, one

Nutritional yeast, one fourth cup

Vegetable broth, four cups

Cauliflower, one large head chopped into florets

Garlic, minced, three tablespoons

Celery, diced, two stalks

Leeks, one pound cleaned and chopped

Olive oil, three tablespoons

Instructions

Fry the cauliflower, garlic, and the leeks in the olive oil in a large soup pot along with the salt, pepper, and the nutmeg. Keep stirring the ingredients often until the leeks begin to wilt. Pour in the bay leaf, nutritional yeast, and the vegetable broth and bring to a boil, then simmer the soup for forty-five minutes until the cauliflower is very tender. Puree the soup very carefully with an immersion blender or a regular blender, then return the pureed soup

to the pot and simmer for fifteen more minutes.

Miso Soup with Shirataki Noodles

Makes two servings

Shopping list

carrot, fresh cilantro, bok choy, green cabbage, pasture-raised chicken breast, miso paste, shirataki noodles, vegetable broth

Ingredients

Sea salt, one teaspoon

Black pepper, one teaspoon

Carrot, one peeled and sliced into ribbons

Cilantro, chopped, one fourth cup

Bok choy, two separated into sections

Green cabbage, shredded, one cup

Chicken breast, pasture-raised, cooked and chopped, one cup

Miso paste, two tablespoons

Shirataki noodles, two cups

Vegetable broth, four cups

Instructions

Put the broth in a large pan over a high heat and cook the noodles, then add in the shredded cabbage and cook this for ten minutes. Turn the heat down and then stir in the miso paste, bok choy, and the chicken. Serve while still hot.

Creamy Shrimp and Cauliflower Soup

Makes four servings

Shopping list

fresh cilantro, aniseeds, leek, riced cauliflower, twelve medium-sized wild-caught shrimp peeled and deveined

Ingredient

Lime juice, two tablespoons

Cilantro, one bunch, chopped

Paprika, one tablespoon

Sea salt, one tablespoon

Black pepper, one tablespoon

Aniseeds, one fourth teaspoon

Coconut milk, two cans

Garlic, minced, two tablespoons

Leek, one large, use the white part only, chopped finely after washing

Olive oil, three tablespoons

Cauliflower rice, one and one half cups

Wild-caught shrimp, twelve medium size

Instructions

Fry the shrimp in the olive oil for three to four minutes on each side, until they turn pink. Take the cooked shrimp out of the pan and set them off to the side. Fry the chopped leek in the oil for two minutes, and then add in the aniseeds and the garlic and fry for three minutes more, stirring often. Then stir in the salt, pepper, paprika, shrimps, and one can of the coconut milk. Mix in the cauliflower and fry for ten minutes until the cauliflower is done.

Remove the shrimp from the mixture and set them to the side while you carefully blend all of the other ingredients until they are creamy and smooth. Chop the shrimp into bite-sized pieces and stir them back into the soup with the chopped cilantro, the lime juice, and the other can of milk.

Cheddar Broccoli Soup

Serves four

Shopping list

goat's milk cheddar cheese, vegetable broth, celery, yellow onion, broccoli florets

Ingredients

Shredded goat's milk cheddar, one cup*

Vegetable broth, two cups

Coconut cream, one cup

Black pepper, one teaspoon

Sea salt, one teaspoon

Garlic, minced, three tablespoons

Celery, diced, two stalks

Yellow onion, one minced

Broccoli florets, two cups

Olive oil, one fourth cup

Instructions

Fry the garlic, celery, onion, and broccoli in the hot olive oil for five minutes, seasoning the mix with the salt and pepper. Pour in the broth, the coconut cream, and three-fourths of the goat cheese into the mix, stirring well to blend. Stir this frequently and cook it for fifteen minutes to allow the cheese to melt. Serve the soup hot with the rest of the shredded cheese as garnish.

*To make this soup in a vegan version, exchange the goat's milk cheese with nutritional yeast.

Cabbage Soup

Makes four servings

Shopping list

vegetable sprouts, white cabbage, celery, carrot, yellow onion

Ingredients

Vegetable sprouts, chopped parsley, or fresh cilantro for garnish for serving

Warm water, five cups

Sea salt, one teaspoon

Black pepper, one teaspoon

Thyme, dried, one teaspoon

White cabbage, one half of one, shredded finely

Ginger, ground, one teaspoon

Celery, one stalk chopped

Carrot, one chopped finely

Yellow onion, one chopped finely

Olive oil, three tablespoons

Instructions

Fry the ginger, celery, carrots, and onions in the hot olive oil in a large soup pot for fifteen minutes, stirring often. Mix in the cabbage with the salt, pepper, and the thyme until well blended and then boil. Pour in the warm water and then simmer for ten minutes. Serve with suggested toppings as desired.

Roasted Veggie Soup

Makes six servings

Shopping list

vegetables broth, green cabbage, onion, fennel, sweet potatoes

Ingredients

Bay leaf, one

Thyme, dried, one teaspoon

Vegetable broth, eight cups

Green cabbage, two pounds chopped in small pieces with the core removed

Onion, one large thinly sliced

Olive oil, one fourth cup

Fennel, one pound, trims off ends and sliced thin

Sweet potatoes, two pounds peeled and cut into one-inch cubes

Instructions

Heat the oven to 450. Place the fennel and sweet potatoes into a bowl and toss them with the black pepper and the sea salt. Put the seasoned veggies on a baking sheet and bake them for forty minutes, stirring once. Put the olive oil into a large soup pot on a high heat and fry the onion for five minutes. Toss in the cabbage and fry for another ten minutes while stirring often. Drop the roasted sweet potato and the fennel into the cabbage mixture, then pour in the broth and stir well and boil. Stir in the thyme and the bay leaf and simmer for fifteen minutes. After fifteen minutes remove the bay leaf and serve.

Vegetable Broth

Makes eight servings

Shopping list

coconut aminos, seaweed, shirataki mushrooms, red cabbage, celery, onion, carrots, kale

Ingredients

Coriander, one bunch fresh

Coconut aminos, one tablespoon

Turmeric, two tablespoons

Peppercorns, one tablespoon

Seaweed, dried, thirty grams

Shirataki mushrooms, one-half cup sliced

Red cabbage, shredded, one cup

Celery, chopped, one cup

Onion, chopped, one cup

Carrots, chopped, one cup

Kale, one cup

Ginger, ground, one tablespoon

Garlic, minced, two tablespoons

Coconut oil, one tablespoon

Sea salt, one teaspoon

Black pepper, one teaspoon

Water, twelve cups

Instructions

Fry the onions, garlic, and celery in the coconut oil in a large soup pot for five minutes, seasoning them with the peppercorns, salt, pepper, turmeric, and ginger. Pour in the water and add in the rest of the ingredients, stirring well, and then boil. Then simmer the soup for one hour. Strain the veggies out of the liquid and discard the veggies. Serve the broth immediately or store it in the refrigerator.

Pumpkin Spice Cauliflower Rice soup

Makes four servings

Shopping list

Rice cauliflower, red onion

<u>**Ingredients**</u>

Pumpkin pie spice, two teaspoons

Coconut milk, one can

Cauliflower rice, four cups

Black pepper, one teaspoon

Sea salt, one teaspoon

Rosemary, ground, one teaspoon

Avocado oil, two tablespoons

Garlic, minced, one tablespoon

Red onion, diced, one half cup

<u>**Instructions**</u>

Fry the garlic and the onion in the hot avocado oil for five minutes. Season them with the pepper, salt, and the rosemary. Stir in the coconut milk, cauliflower rice, and the pumpkin spice and boil. Then simmer the soup for twenty minutes and serve warm.

Lemon Chicken Kale Soup

Serves six

<u>**Shopping list**</u>

Parmigiano Reggiano cheese, kale, pasture-raised chicken breast, vegetable broth, celery, onion

<u>**Ingredients**</u>

Parmigiano Reggiano cheese for serving

Black pepper, one teaspoon

Sea salt, one teaspoon

Lemon juice, two tablespoons

Kale, two bunches washed and chopped

Pasture-raised chicken breast, one cup cooked and cubed

Dijon mustard, one half teaspoon

Balsamic vinegar, one teaspoon

Vegetable broth, five cups

Celery, two stalks minced

Garlic, minced, four tablespoons

Onion, one medium-sized diced finely

Olive oil, three tablespoons

<u>**Instructions**</u>

Fry the celery, garlic, and the onion along with the salt and pepper for five minutes. Mix in the kale, Dijon mustard, and the chicken with the lemon juice and cook this mixture for another five minutes. Then pour in the vegetables broth and the balsamic vinegar and boil, then simmer for forty minutes and serve.

Celery Soup

Serves four

Shopping list

one lemon, fresh parsley, vegetable broth, onion, celery, celery root

Ingredients

Parsley, three tablespoons chopped for garnish

Lemon, one

Vegetable broth, three cups

Black pepper, one teaspoon

Sea salt, one teaspoon

Rosemary, dried, one teaspoon

Onion, minced, one fourth cup

Celery, two stalks cut into cubes

Celery root, one pound cut into cubes

Olive oil, three tablespoons

Instructions

Fry the onion, celery, and celery root in the hot olive oil in a large soup pot with the pepper, salt, and rosemary to season. Cook all of this for five minutes, stirring often. Slice the lemon thinly and add it to the pot, and then pour in the vegetable broth and boil, then simmer for thirty minutes. Pour one-fourth of the soup into a blender and blend it until it is creamy and smooth and then pour it into a serving bowl, then repeat with the remainder of the soup. Scoop the soup into serving bowls and then garnish with the chopped parsley.

Mushroom Soup

Serves two

Shopping list

onion, hemp seed hearts, mushrooms

Ingredients

Thyme, dried, one half teaspoon

Black pepper, one half teaspoon

Sea salt, one half teaspoon

Onion, minced, one tablespoon

Hemp seed hearts, one half cup

Water, one cup

Mushrooms, fresh, three cups without stems

Instructions

Keep one-half cup of the mushrooms, chop them, and set them to the side. Put the salt, pepper, thyme, onions, hemp seed hearts, water, and the rest of the mushrooms into your blender and then blend all of the ingredients together until they are creamy and smooth. If it is needed, add in a bit more water. Pour the blended soup ingredients into a pot and warm over a low heat for ten minutes, stirring often. Garnish with the chopped mushrooms and serve.

Fall Harvest Vegetable Soup

Makes six servings

Shopping list

sweet potato, white onion, celery, radishes, carrots

Ingredients

Water, four cups

Sea salt, one teaspoon

Black pepper, one teaspoon

Curry powder, one teaspoon

Olive oil, one tablespoon

Sweet potato, one medium-sized

White onion, one medium-sized

Celery, three stalks

Radishes, five

Carrots, two medium

Garlic, minced, four tablespoons

Ginger, ground, one teaspoon

<u>Instructions</u>

Peel the onion, sweet potato, and carrots and chop everything into bite-sized pieces, including the celery. Fry the garlic, ginger, and onion in a large soup pot in the olive oil for five minutes. Mix in the carrots, celery, and the sweet potato and cover all of this with water and boil. Stir in the salt, pepper, and curry and let the soup simmer for thirty minutes and serve.

Chapter 11
Dessert Recipes

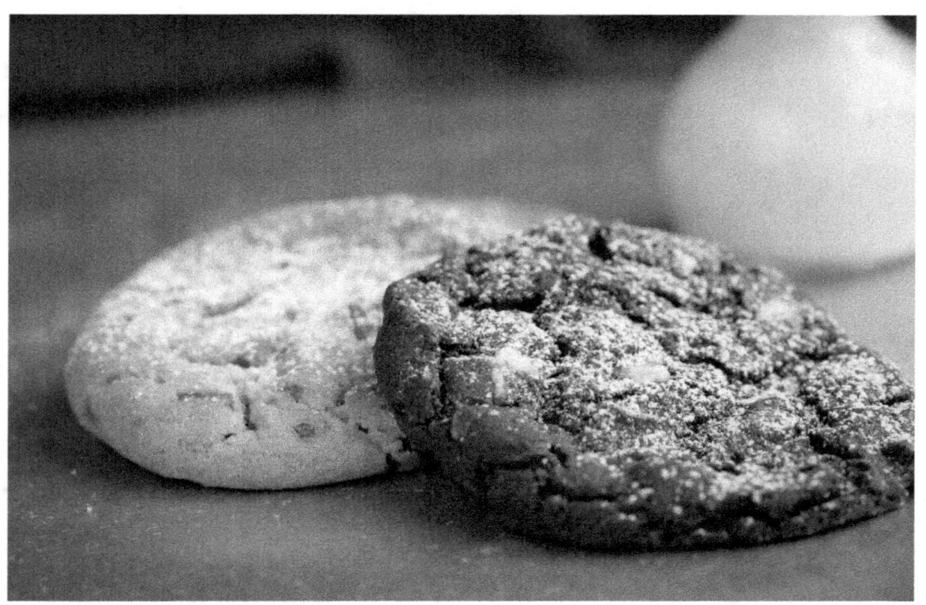

Coconut Chocolate Ice Pops

Makes six to eight pops

<u>**Shopping list**</u>

 bittersweet chocolate, shredded coconut

<u>**Ingredients**</u>

Coconut oil, one tablespoon

Bittersweet Chocolate, seventy percent or higher, one-half cup chopped

Stevie, twelve drops

Shredded coconut, unsweetened, one half cup

Coconut milk, two cans

<u>**Instructions**</u>

Blend together the stevia, shredded coconut, and the coconut milk in a large pot over a low heat. Stir three-fourths of the chocolate into the pan, stirring continuously until the chocolate is melted. Take the pot off the stove and let the mixture cool to room temperature. Then pour the batter into popsicle molds and freeze for three hours. After three hours, mix the leftover amount of the chocolate together with the coconut oil in a little pot over a low heat until they are melted and well mixed. Remove the pops from the molds and coat them with the coconut oil chocolate mixture

Chocolate Snack Cake

Makes one eight-inch round cake

Shopping list

 bittersweet chocolate, coconut cream, pastured eggs, almond flour

Ingredients

Vanilla extract, one teaspoon

Bittersweet chocolate, two tablespoons

Coconut cream, unsweetened, one third cup

Pastured eggs, three

Sea salt, one half teaspoon

Baking powder, aluminum-free, one teaspoon

Natural cocoa powder, unsweetened, one fourth cup

Erythritol, two-thirds cup

Almond flour, one cup

Olive oil, one fourth cup

Spray olive oil

<u>**Instructions**</u>

Heat the oven to 350. Use the spray oil to grease an eight-inch round cake pan and set it to the side. Use a large mixing bowl to blend together the sea salt, baking powder, cocoa powder, erythritol, and the almond flour. Use a smaller mixing bowl to blend the coconut cream and the eggs. Then melt the vanilla and olive oil with the chocolate over a low heat or in the microwave until the chocolate is melted and all of the ingredients are creamy and smooth. Let the chocolate mixture cool for five minutes and then blend it in to the mixture of coconut cream. Pour the blended ingredients from the small bowl into the ingredients in the large bowl and stir gently but thoroughly to blend all of the ingredients together. Pour the batter into the spray oiled cake pan and bake for thirty-five minutes. Cool the cake to room temperature before serving.

Spice Cookies

Makes twelve cookies

<u>Shopping list</u>

A2 protein butter, coconut flour, walnuts

<u>Ingredients</u>

Sea salt, one fourth teaspoon

Vanilla extract, one half teaspoon

Almond extract, one half teaspoon

Butter, A2 protein only, one-fourth cup softened to room temperature

Coconut flour, one fourth cup

Monk fruit sweetener, one half cup

Cloves, ground, one eighth teaspoon

Cinnamon, ground, one half teaspoon

Nutmeg, ground, one half teaspoon

Walnuts, toasted, one cup

<u>Instructions</u>

Heat the oven to 325. Lay parchment paper on two baking sheets. Chop the walnuts finely and then mix them with the cloves, cinnamon, and the nutmeg. Blend these with the coconut flour and the erythritol until all of the ingredients are well mixed. Stir in the softened butter with the sea salt, almond extract, and the vanilla extract and keep mixing the dough gently until you have formed a soft ball of dough. Divide the ball of dough into twelve equal-sized portions and then roll each of these into a ball. Set them on the baking sheets and flatten them slightly. Bake the cookies, one baking sheet at a time on the middle oven rack, for fifteen minutes. Then let the cookies thaw for thirty minutes before you move them off the baking sheet.

Sweet Potato Cinnamon Blondies

Makes twelve

<u>Shopping list</u>

coconut flour, almond flour, pastured eggs, sweet potato

Ingredients

Sea salt, one half teaspoon

Vanilla extract, one teaspoon

Cloves, ground, one fourth teaspoon

Cinnamon, ground, one teaspoon

Baking soda, one half teaspoon

Coconut flour, three tablespoons

Almond flour, two cups

Pastured eggs, three

Coconut milk, one cup

Sweet potato puree, one half cup

Monk fruit sweetener, one third cup

Coconut oil, one-third cup softened to room temperature

Olive oil spray

Instructions

Heat the oven to 350. Use the spray oil to grease an eight by eight-inch baking dish and then set it to the side. Cream together the coconut oil and the monk fruit sweetener in a large bowl until they are creamy and smooth. Blend in the eggs, coconut milk, and the sweet potato puree. Mix in the sea salt, vanilla extract, cinnamon, cloves, baking soda, and the two flours and stir until the ingredients are all well blended. Press the batter gently but firmly into the greased baking dish and bake this for forty-five minutes. Cool the pan of blondies to room temperature before trying to slice it.

Olive Oil Rosemary Cake

Serves twelve slices

Shopping list

one orange, almond flour

Ingredients

CAKE

Olive oil, two-thirds cup

Lemon juice, two tablespoons

Baking powder, two teaspoons

Xylitol, one cup

Rosemary, dried, one tablespoon

Orange zest, two tablespoons

Almond flour, one and one half cups

Olive oil spray

<u>SYRUP</u>

Xylitol, four tablespoons

Lemon juice, two tablespoons

Water, one half cup

<u>Instructions</u>

Use the spray oil to grease an eight by eight-inch baking dish. Mix together the rosemary, orange zest, and the almond flour until they are well mixed in a large size mixing bowl. Stir in the lemon juice, baking powder, and the xylitol until well blended. Then stir in the eggs and olive oil until thoroughly mixed together. Place the batter in the baking dish and bake the cake for thirty minutes, then leave it in the baking dish to cool. Prepare the syrup recipe while the cake is cooling by warming in a small pan all of the syrup ingredients over a low heat and then boil for five minutes. Poke holes in the cake with a kebab stick and pour the syrup over the cake and let it cool.

Mint Chocolate Chip Avocado Ice Cream

Makes six servings

<u>Shopping list</u>

extra-dark chocolate chips, avocados, dark chocolate baking bar, coffee powder, coconut cream

<u>Ingredients</u>

Chocolate chips, extra dark, sugar-free, one half cup

Stevia, ten drops

Avocados, two peeled and pitted

Vanilla extract, one teaspoon

Dark chocolate, sugar-free, three ounces chopped

Cocoa powder, unsweetened, two tablespoons

Coffee powder, instant, one teaspoon

Erythritol, three-fourths cup

Coconut cream, one can

Instructions

Warm the cocoa powder, coffee powder, erythritol, and the coconut milk in a pan over a low heat, stirring constantly until they are well blended. Take the pan off the stove and stir in the chopped chocolate until it is melted and mixed in. Blend in the stevia, avocado pulp, and the vanilla extract until all of the ingredients are well blended. Stir in the chocolate chips and put the mixture into a freezer-safe bowl and freeze for four hours before serving.

Chocolate Almond Butter Cake

Serves one

Shopping list

almond butter, grass-fed ghee, coconut cream, pastured egg

Ingredients

Almond butter, smooth, one tablespoon

Grass-fed ghee, one teaspoon

Vanilla extract, one half teaspoon

Coconut cream, one tablespoon

Pastured egg, one

Baking powder, aluminum-free, one fourth teaspoon

Xylitol, two tablespoons

Cocoa powder, unsweetened, two tablespoons

<u>**Instructions**</u>

Blend the baking powder, xylitol, and the cocoa powder in a large-sized mixing bowl. Stir in the vanilla, coconut cream, and the egg until the entire ingredients are blended well. Use spray oil to grease a large coffee mug and pour the cake batter into it. Microwave the mug for one minute twenty seconds and then drizzle the softened almond butter over the top of the cake.

Rice Pudding

Makes four servings

<u>**Shopping list**</u>

pastured egg, grass-fed ghee, coconut milk, arrowroot powder, shirataki rice

<u>**Ingredients**</u>

Pastured egg, one

Cocoa powder, one fourth cup

Vanilla extract, one tablespoon

Xylitol, one cup

Ghee, one teaspoon

Coconut milk, three and one half cups

Arrowroot powder, five tablespoons

Shirataki rice, two cups

Olive oil spray

Instructions

Heat the oven to 350. Rinse the shirataki rice and set it to the side. Place the cocoa powder, coffee powder, xylitol, and the coconut milk in a pan over a medium heat until it is warm and well blended. Take the pan from the stove and blend in the chopped chocolate. In another bowl, blend the avocados and the vanilla extract until they are smooth and creamy. Blend in the rice along with the chocolate chips and refrigerate this for one hour and then serve.

Gingersnap Cookies

Makes twenty-four

Shopping list

almond flour, pastured egg, Italian butter

Ingredients

Allspice, ground, one fourth teaspoon

Cinnamon, ground, one fourth teaspoon

Cloves, ground, one fourth teaspoon

Nutmeg, ground, one fourth teaspoon

Ginger, ground, one teaspoon

Baking soda, one teaspoon

Sea salt, one fourth teaspoon

Almond flour, two cups

Vanilla extract, one teaspoon

Pastured egg, one

Erythritol, one cup

Italian butter, unsalted, one-fourth cup at room temperature

<u>Instructions</u>

Heat the oven to 350. Blend well together in a large size mixing bowl the allspice, cloves, cinnamon, nutmeg, ginger, baking soda, salt, and the flour until all of the ingredients are well blended. Use a small-sized mixing bowl to cream together the vanilla extract, egg, erythritol, and the butter and then pour this into the large mixing bowl and mix together well. Use a tablespoon to measure out the cookies and then bake them on a spray-oiled baking sheet for fifteen minutes. Let the cookies cool to room temperature.

Lemon Bars

Makes fifteen bars

Shopping list

arrowroot flour, one lemon, pastured eggs, arrowroot flour, Tigernut flour, almond flour, Italian butter

Ingredients

FILLING

Arrowroot flour, two tablespoons

Monk fruit sweetener, one half cup

Lemon zest, one tablespoon

Lemon juice, one half cup

Pastured eggs, six

TOPPING

Lemon zest, one tablespoon

Monk fruit sweetener, two tablespoons

Sea salt, one fourth teaspoon

Arrowroot flour, one fourth cup

Tigernut flour, three-fourths cup

Almond flour, three-fourths cup

Italian butter, unsalted, twelve tablespoons softened to room temperature

Instructions

Heat the oven to 350. Mix all of the topping ingredients together well until they make a mass of wet crumbs, then press them into a spray-oiled thirteen by nine-inch baking pan, on the bottom only. Bake this for twenty minutes. Then blend well together all of the ingredients listed for the filling. When the crust has finished baking, let it cool for thirty minutes and then pour on the filling, then bake this for fifteen more minutes. Let the lemon bars cool down to room temperature before slicing it.

Ginger Sheet Cake

<u>Shopping list</u>

coconut milk, pastured eggs, A2 protein butter, almond flour, cassava flour, confectioner's

erythritol, cream cheese

<u>Ingredients</u>

<u>BUTTERMILK</u>

Apple cider vinegar, one tablespoon

Coconut milk, unsweetened, three-fourths cup

<u>GINGER CAKE</u>

Buttermilk mixture

Vanilla extract, one teaspoon

Pastured eggs, two

Erythritol, one half cup

Butter, A2 protein, unsalted, one-fourth cup softened to room temperature

Sea salt, one fourth teaspoon

Baking powder, one half teaspoon

Baking soda, three-fourths teaspoon

Pumpkin pie spice, two teaspoons

Ginger, ground, two teaspoons

Almond flour, one third cup

Cassava flour, three-fourths cup

CREAM CHEESE ICING

Cinnamon, ground, one tablespoon

Vanilla extract, one teaspoon

Confectioner's erythritol, three-fourths cup

Cream cheese, full fat, four ounces softened to room temperature

Butter, A2 protein, unsalted, four ounces softened to room temperature

Instructions

Heat the oven to 300 and set the oven rack in the middle of the oven. Use olive oil spray oil to grease a thirteen by nine-inch baking dish. Mix together the apple cider vinegar and the coconut milk in a small cup and set it off to the side. Blend together in a large bowl, the salt, baking powder, baking soda, pumpkin pie spice, ginger, and the flour until blended well. In another smaller mixing bowl, cream together the vanilla, sugar, butter, and the eggs until well blended and creamy. Then stir in the buttermilk and mix well. Pour the small bowl ingredients into the large bowl ingredients and fold gently to mix together well. Put the batter into the spray oiled thirteen by nine-inch baking dish and baked the cake for forty minutes. Make the cream cheese icing while the cake is in the oven by first creaming together the cream cheese and the butter until they are well blended. Then blend in the vanilla extract and the confectioner's erythritol. The icing needs to be just thin enough so that you can spread it on the cake. When the ginger cake has cooled completely, spread the cream cheese icing over the entire top and then sprinkle on the cinnamon for garnish.

Summertime Strawberry Shortcake

Makes eight servings

Shopping list

fresh strawberries, grass-fed heavy cream, arrowroot starch, tigernut flour, coconut flour, one lemon, coconut cream, pastured eggs, Italian butter

Ingredients

TOPPING

Strawberries, fresh, one quart hulled and slice

Vanilla extract, one half teaspoon

Monk fruit sweetener, one tablespoon

Grass-fed heavy cream, one cup

CAKE

Baking soda, three-fourths teaspoon

Sea salt, one half teaspoon

Arrowroot starch, three tablespoons

Tigernut flour, one third cup

Coconut flour, one third cup

Vanilla extract, one half teaspoon

Lemon zest, one tablespoon

Coconut cream, one half cup

Pastured eggs, three

Monk fruit sweetener, one fourth cup

Italian butter, eight tablespoons softened to room temperature

Instructions

Heat the oven to 350. Use spray oil to grease an eight-inch round cake pan. Cream together the sweetener and the butter until creamy and fluffy. The blend in the vanilla extract, lemon zest, coconut cream, and the eggs until well blended. In a different sized mixing bowl, blend together the baking soda, sea salt, arrowroot starch, Tigernut flour, and the coconut flour. Pour in the bowl of butter mixture and blend all of the ingredients together until they are well mixed. Put the batter into the spray, oiled eight-inch pan and bake the cake for thirty minutes. Let the shortcake cool in the pan for thirty minutes and then turn it out onto a cooling rack. Beat together the vanilla extract, monk fruit sweetener, and the cream until the mixture makes soft peaks. Spread this topping on top of the cake and then decorate the cake with the strawberries.

Candy Crunch Bars

Makes twenty-four bars

Shopping list

millet, sesame seeds, hemp hearts, dark chocolate baking bar

Ingredients

Sea salt, one half teaspoon

Puffed millet, one and one half cups

Sesame seeds, one fourth cup

Hemp hearts, one fourth cup

Dark chocolate, twenty-four ounces in pieces

Instructions

Melt the dark chocolate until it is creamy and smooth. Blend the sesame seeds with the puffed millet and take out two tablespoons to set to the side for the topping. Stir the puffed millet and the sesame seeds into the melted chocolate. Use olive oil spray oil to spray oil a thirteen by nine-inch baking dish and then carefully press flat the mixture into the bottom of the baking dish. Sprinkle the reserved puffed millet and the sesame seeds on the top, and then put the dish in the refrigerator to chill for one hour before slicing it.

Berry Birthday Cake

Serves four to six

Shopping list

dark chocolate chips, cacao butter, fresh berries of choice, coconut cream, dark chocolate baking bar, pastured eggs, cacao powder, almond flour

Ingredients

GLAZE

Monk fruit sweetener, two teaspoons

Vanilla extract, one half teaspoon

Dark chocolate chips, one half cup

Cacao butter, one ounce

DECORATION

Berries of your choice, one cup when in season

FILLING

Vanilla extract, one half teaspoon

Monk fruit sweetener, two teaspoons

Coconut cream, one cup

<u>**CAKE**</u>

Vanilla extract, one teaspoon

Dark chocolate bar, three tablespoons

Coconut cream, full fat, one third cup

Pastured eggs, three

Sea salt, one half teaspoon

Monk fruit sweetener, three tablespoons

Olive oil, one fourth cup

Cacao powder, one fourth cup

Baking powder, one teaspoon

Almond flour, one cup

<u>**Instructions**</u>

Heat the oven to 350. Use olive oil spray oil to grease two eight-inch cake pans and set them off to the side. Make the cakes by blending together the salt, sweetener, baking powder, cacao, and the flour until well blended. Then stir in gently the coconut cream and the eggs until the batter is creamy and smooth. Then blend in the olive oil, vanilla, and the melted chocolate and mix all of the ingredients together well. Pour the cake batter into the two greased cake pans and bake them for twenty-five minutes. Let the cakes layers cool completely before turning them out onto a flat surface like a dinner plate. Carefully slice each layer in half through the middle. Make the glaze by adding all of the ingredients to a small pan and warming them over a low heat stirring continuously until all of the ingredients are well blended. Prepare the cream by whipping together the vanilla extract, sweetener, and the heavy cream until it makes solid peaks. Set down one cake layer on a serving plate and then top it with cream, a few berries, and then more cream. Put on the next cake layer and keep repeating all of the layers until all of the ingredients are sued, and the cake is completely put together.

Chocolate Chip Cookies

Shopping list

dark chocolate chips, almond flour, pastured eggs

Ingredients

Chocolate chips, dark chocolate, one cup

Sea salt, one half teaspoon

Baking soda, one teaspoon

Almond flour, four cups

Vanilla extract, two teaspoons

Pastured eggs, two

Monk fruit sweetener, six tablespoons

Coconut oil, four tablespoons

Instructions

Heat the oven to 375. Use olive oil spray to grease a baking sheet. Mix the monk fruit sweetener and the coconut oil until they are well blended. Then cream in the vanilla and the eggs. Then stir in the salt, baking soda, and the flour and mix well until you have a smooth batter, and then gently fold in the chips of chocolate. Make one inch sized balls of dough and flatten them slightly, then bake the cookies for ten minutes and cool them on a wire

rack.

Chapter 12
The Plant Paradox Way Of Life

So now you have your lists of foods to eat and foods to avoid, and some of the recipes that will use these foods in flavorful and delicious ways. You know what to look for in the foods that you buy for your meals. You also know what foods to keep on hand to plan meals around, and how to eat some of the foods that contain lectin by removing the part of the food that contains the lectin.

Now it is time to put all of this together in a sensible eating plan that will change your life forever. If you use the right kinds of foods in a healthy eating plan, then you will lose weight and feel great.

You will begin the Plant Paradox diet by doing the three-day cleanses. This part is mandatory, and you may not skip it, because it is necessary for your body to clean out all of the toxins that have been building up over the years. This might not clean out all of your built-up toxins, but it will provide a good beginning, and the diet will take care of the rest. So to begin the diet, you will give up the following foods completely:

Soy	Eggs	Corn
Seeds	Sugar	Dairy
Tubers	Canola	Fruit
Grains	Pseudo-grains	Inflammatory oils
Nightshade plants	Farm animal proteins	

If you feel like you need a snack during this phase, you may use the following foods for snack items: avocado, approved nuts, leafy greens, olive oil, and lemon juice. Sleep is important, preferably seven or eight hours every night, because your body needs time to adjust and sleep will help with this. Keep your protein to no more than eight ounces each day and no more than four ounces in any one meal, but you can eat as many of the vegetables on the 'yes' list as you would like to eat. For all of the menu suggestions, the recipes are found in this book.

THREE-DAY DETOX DIET

Make up the Breakfast Salad Dressing, Nutty Green Salad Dressing, and the nut Mix and have them ready for this week.

DAY ONE

Breakfast	Green Ginger Smoothie
Lunch	Nutty Green Salad
Dinner	Mushroom and Sage Soup

DAY TWO

Breakfast	Green Ginger Smoothie
Lunch	Cauliflower Rice
Dinner	Avocado and Salmon Bowl

DAY THREE

Breakfast	Green Ginger Smoothie

Lunch	Breakfast Salad

PHASE TWO EATING PLAN

When you complete the Three-Day Cleanse, then you will move right into Phase Two. You will remain on Phase Two for the next six weeks. Here are some sample menus for Phase Two, and all of the recipes are located in this book.

DAY ONE

Breakfast	Almond Muffins
Lunch	Chicken Salad
Dinner	Veggie Noodle Bake

DAY TWO

Breakfast	Baked Avocado Cups with Pesto
Lunch	Portobello Mushroom Pizza
Dinner	Chicken and Veggies

DAY THREE

Breakfast	Green Egg Muffins
Lunch	Bok Choy with Shrimp

| Dinner | Swedish Meatballs |

PHASE THREE EATING PLAN

This is the final phase of the Plant Paradox diet, and it is meant to be the way that you will eat for the remainder of your life.

__DAY ONE__

Breakfast	Carrot Cake Muffins
Lunch	Baked Artichoke Hearts
Dinner	Beef and Mushrooms

__DAY TWO__

Breakfast	Plantain Pancakes
Lunch	Collard Wrapped Burritos
Dinner	Shrimp Risotto

__DAY THREE__

Breakfast	Cheesy Cauliflower Cups
Lunch	Sesame Noodle Salad
Dinner	Chicken Seaweed Wraps

Remember that any smoothie recipe can take the place of a meal if you are just not feeling that hungry at mealtime, and a smoothie makes a great snack any time outside of the detox phase. In Phase Two, feel free to add in a few desserts because a sweet treat now and then can keep you happy and motivated. And if you fall of the diet wagon at any point, just start again fresh the next day. If you have missed several days, you might want to start over with the detox phase, but don't beat yourself up since we are all human. Do your best, and don't be afraid to try new foods, and you will be successful.

Conclusion

Thank you for making it through to the end of *Lectin Free Diet: Healthy Foods from another Point of View with Recipes and Weekly Menu* by Igea Bardo, let's hope it was informative and able to provide you with all of the tools you need to achieve your goals whatever they may be.

The next step is to make the decision to switch to a lectin free life and do yourself the favor of removing the harmful lectins from your food and your life. You owe it to yourself to eat a diet that is free of lectins and full of the healthy foods that will help you to lose weight, decrease inflammation and skin irritations, and just generally make you feel better so that you can live the life that you want to live.

Try the delicious recipes in this book and then experiment with some of your own, using the ones here as a guide. I would especially recommend that you try the desserts, because even a lectin-free diet can taste great.

Finally, if you found this book useful in any way, a review on Amazon is always appreciated! Write your email if you want to be warned in advance of new books coming out.

Igea Bardo

www.ingramcontent.com/pod-product-compliance
Lightning Source LLC
Chambersburg PA
CBHW070703250726
48662CB00001B/230